Tracheostomy and Artificial Ventilation

in the treatment of respiratory failure

Tracheostomy and Artificial Ventilation

in the treatment of respiratory failure

Edited by Stanley A. Feldman
Consultant Anaesthetist, Westminster Hospital, London

and Brian E. Crawley
Consultant Anaesthetist, Canterbury Group of Hospitals

Third Edition

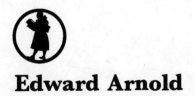

Edward Arnold

© Edward Arnold (Publishers) Ltd, 1977

First published 1967
by Edward Arnold (Publishers) Ltd
25 Hill Street, London W1X 8LL

Second edition, 1971
Third edition, 1977

British Library Cataloguing in Publication Data
Tracheostomy and artificial ventilation
  in the treatment of respiratory failure.
  —3rd ed.
  1. Respiratory insufficiency
  I. Feldman, Stanley Anthony II. Crawley,
  Brian Edward
  616.2′004′6   RC732

  ISBN 0-7131-4288-X
  ISBN 0-7131-4289-8 Pbk

Filmset in 'Monophoto' Baskerville 10 on 11 pt and
printed in Great Britain by
Richard Clay (The Chaucer Press), Ltd,
Bungay, Suffolk

Contributors

B. E. Crawley, MB, BS, FFARCS, DA
Consultant Anaesthetist, Canterbury Group of Hospitals

A. Doughty, MB, BS, FFARCS
Consultant Anaesthetist, Kingston Hospital, Surrey

P. A. Emerson, MA, MD, FRCP, FACP (Hon)
Consultant Physician, Westminster Hospital, London

S. Farquharson, MB, BS, FFARCS, DA
Consultant Anaesthetist, Norfolk and Norwich Hospital

S. A. Feldman, BSc, MB, BS, FFARCS, DA
Consultant Anaesthetist, Westminster Hospital, London

H. Gaya, MB, ChB, MRCPath.
Reader in Bacteriology, St Mary's Hospital Medical School, London

W. J. Glover, MB, BCh, BAO, FFARCS, DObstRCOG
Consultant Anaesthetist, Hospital for Sick Children, Great Ormond
Street, London

M. Green, MA, BSc, BM, MRCP
Consultant Physician, St Bartholomew's and Brompton Hospitals,
London

Julian M. Leigh, MD, FFARCS
Consultant Anaesthetist and Director, Intensive Care Unit, Royal Surrey
County Hospital, Guildford

H. F. Seeley, MA, MSc, MB, BS, FFARCS
Lecturer in Anaesthetics, Westminster Hospital Medical School, London

Miss G. Tobin, SRN
Formerly Sister-in-Charge, Intensive Care Unit, Westminster Hospital,
London

with the assistance of
Miss J. Boorman, SRN
and
Mrs. V. Johnston

Preface

When this book was first published in 1967, few hospitals had specialized intensive care units. Today there is hardly a hospital that has not either a special intensive care unit or separate intensive therapy beds. The technical sophistication of these units varies enormously from those with on-line computerized monitoring and real time data display of vital functions to simple units run by a competent doctor together with well trained nurses. It is evident that in spite of all the technological advances the most important factor in determining the success of the treatment remains that of a sound understanding of the problems involved and a high level of patient care by the nursing staff. It is to this end that special training courses have been organized for nurses working in the intensive care units. It is hoped that this book, which draws largely on the practical experience of doctors involved in this form of therapy, will help to supplement this training, as well as to fulfil the needs of the medical student or doctor who wishes to enquire further into the indications for and the benefits and limitations of tracheostomy and artificial ventilation.

The third edition of this book has seen a major revision of all the chapters as befits a book on such a rapidly developing subject. Completely new chapters on parenteral nutrition, oxygen therapy, nursing care and physiotherapy of patients receiving artificial ventilation have been introduced. A ten-year review of the changing pattern observed in the ICU of one district general hospital is presented in the final chapter which gives an historical perspective of the major changes that have occurred, as well as an indication of the new problems that are emerging.

It is hoped that doctors in all disciplines as well as nurses and students will find the information helps them to understand the problems that occur when treating seriously ill patients by means of a tracheostomy or by artificial ventilation.

SAF
BEC

Acknowledgements

The authors are indebted to the Staff of the Intensive Care Unit of Westminster Hospital, and to Sister Boorman and the Staff of the Kent and Canterbury Hospital Intensive Care Unit, who have helped in the preparation of the third edition of this book.

Contents

Preface vii

Acknowledgements viii

Introduction x

1 Pathophysiology of Respiratory Failure
        P. A. Emerson and M. Green 1

2 Respiratory Failure—Diagnosis and Treatment
        P. A. Emerson and M. Green 8

3 Indications for Tracheostomy and Laryngotomy *S. A. Feldman* 22

4 Indications for Artificial Ventilation
        P. A. Emerson and M. Green 28

5 Physiological Effects of Tracheostomy and Artificial Respiration
           S. A. Feldman 35

6 Oxygen Therapy—Theory and Practice *J. M. Leigh* 41

7 Technique of Tracheostomy *B. E. Crawley* 53

8 Complications of Tracheostomy *B. E. Crawley* 64

9 Management of a Tracheostomy *B. E. Crawley* 73

10 Automatic Ventilators *B. E. Crawley* 86

11 Management of Artificial Ventilation
       B. E. Crawley and H. Seeley 100

  Appendix 1: Nursing Care of a Ventilated Patient
    Miss G. Tobin, with assistance of *Miss J. Boorman* 115

  Appendix 2: Physiotherapy Care of a Ventilated Patient
        Mrs. V. Johnston 124

12 Parenteral Nutrition *S. Farquharson* 129

13 Artificial Ventilation, Tracheostomy and Prolonged Intubation
  in Infancy *W. J. Glover* 143

14 Measurements during Artificial Ventilation and their
  Significance *S. A. Feldman* 161

15 Infection—Epidemiology, Prevention and Treatment *H. Gaya* 170

16 Intensive Care in a District General Hospital *A. Doughty* 189

  Index 209

Introduction

Each year more and more patients are being treated by tracheostomy and artificial ventilation. The care of these very ill patients places a heavy burden upon the hospital as the treatment of every patient involves a large number of highly trained staff, elaborate machinery and the expenditure of much time and money. In many hospitals the demand for this form of treatment is so great that beds have been set aside in special 'Respiratory Units' and 'Intensive Care Units'. The centralization of experienced medical, nursing and auxiliary personnel within these units increases the efficiency with which these patients can be treated. It also prevents the dispersal and reduplication of the expensive and delicate machinery that is required, not only for the treatment of the patients, but also for monitoring their progress.

It is therefore all the more surprising that this expanding sphere of medical treatment, with its exacting and expensive requirements, should receive so little attention in the training programme of most hospitals. This is principally because the responsibility for the care of these patients is divided between the physicians, the anaesthetists and the ENT surgeons.

This book is presented in an effort to overcome these barriers and to offer the reader the accumulated experience of all those doctors who are intimately concerned in this form of treatment for respiratory failure. The emphasis of the book is essentially on the practical aspects of this form of therapy and the means of recognizing and avoiding the many pitfalls and complications that can occur. If this treatment is to succeed in these desperately ill patients, then every effort must be made to avoid any possible complication and to recognize the very first warning sign that all is not well. Only by this means can the morbidity and mortality, associated with the tracheostomy and artificial ventilation itself, be reduced to a minimum.

Chapter 1

Pathophysiology of Respiratory Failure

In an average man at rest the lungs transfer over 300 litres of oxygen from the air to the blood and eliminate about 240 litres of carbon dioxide every 24 hours. When the lungs are unable to exchange sufficient gas volumes, the amounts of these gases in the blood alter and at a certain level respiratory failure is said to be present. The term **respiratory insufficiency** may be used to describe the condition in which the blood gases are normal at rest but become abnormal on exercise. The normal level of arterial oxygen tension (Pa_{O_2}) is 95 mm Hg (or 12·7 kPa*) (range 80–100 mm Hg or 10·7–13·3 kPa) and of carbon dioxide tension (Pa_{CO_2}) is 40 mm Hg or 5·3 kPa (range 36–44 mm Hg or 4·8–5·9 kPa). The levels of blood gases at which diagnosis of **respiratory failure** is made must be somewhat arbitrary. However, it is now generally agreed that respiratory failure is present if the Pa_{O_2} falls below 60 mm Hg (8·0 kPa) or the Pa_{CO_2} increases above 50 mm Hg (6·7 kPa) when a patient is breathing air at rest and at sea level.

The function of the lungs is to exchange gases between the external environment (that is, the atmosphere) and the internal environment (that is, the blood stream). It is essential that there should be a correspondence between the ventilation of the lungs with air and the perfusion of the lungs with blood. Therefore there are three aspects to any consideration of respiratory failure:

1. The ventilation of lungs with air.
2. The perfusion of the lungs with blood.
3. The relationship of ventilation to perfusion.

1. Ventilation of the lungs

Pulmonary ventilation may be impaired not only in amount but also in the evenness of its distribution. Reduction in amount occurs when there is disordered function of the respiratory centre or central nervous system and in diseases affecting the respiratory muscles or the nerves supplying them. It also occurs in disorders of the chest wall and the pleura and when there is loss of lung tissue; for instance, with lobar collapse or a large space-occupying lesion in the lung.

The ordered distribution of ventilation is particularly disturbed when

* The unit of pressure measurement adopted in the Système Internationale (SI units) is the kilopascal: 1 kPa unit = 7·5 mm Hg.

there is generalized lung disease. It is useful to divide the disturbances of lung function in generalized lung disease into two categories: **obstructive lung disease** and **restrictive lung disease**.

Obstructive lung disease

This occurs when the passage of air down the tracheobronchial tree is impaired by narrowing of airways. The main resistance to air flow lies in the larger airways (generations 1–12) and so when these are narrowed as in asthma or severe chronic bronchitis, characteristic features are seen. The patient is dyspnoeic and often wheezy. Lung function tests reveal a reduction in **peak expiratory flow rate** (PEFR), conveniently measured with a Wright Peak Flow Meter. The volume of air which can be expired in 1 second (forced expiratory volume in 1 second, FEV_1) is reduced both in absolute terms and as a percentage of forced vital capacity ($FEV_1/FVC\%$). Airway resistance measured in a body plethysmograph or with an oesophageal balloon, is increased (normal < 2 cm H_2O/l/sec or < 0.2 kPa * l^{-1} s^{-1}). If lung function apparatus is not available, a simple clinical test is to measure the number of seconds taken to expire a maximum vital capacity (forced expiratory time, FET). An even simpler and cruder test is to see whether the patient can, with his mouth open, blow out a match.

Frequently the smaller airways (less than 2 mm diameter; generations 12–22) are narrowed, as well as the large airways, and some may even close completely. This results in a reduction of the vital capacity (VC). Lung volumes can be measured in a body plethysmograph or by helium dilution; they may show an increase in total lung capacity (TLC) and residual volumes (RV) (see Fig. 1.1). Sometimes air trapping occurs due to collapse of a larger air passage preventing the escape of air in the smaller passages and in the alveoli distal to the obstruction. This is indicated by an increase in the ratio of RV to TLC. In early bronchitis there may be damage to small, but not large, airways with no detectable change in conventional lung function tests. For this reason the small airways have been called the silent zone. Despite this they are crucial to the ordered distribution of ventilation through the lungs, and damage to them causes severe mismatch of ventilation to perfusion (see p. 4).

Restrictive lung disease

This occurs when there is disease in the parenchyma of the lungs which causes the lung tissue to become stiff and resistant to stretch. It occurs in pulmonary fibrosis which is a result of inflammatory changes. These may be due to fibrosing alveolitis, some of the collagen diseases or drugs such as bleomycin. The FEV_1 and FVC are reduced but the FEV_1/FVC ratio is normal or high. PEFR is partly a function of lung volume and so may also be reduced. Airway resistance is normal but the efficiency of transfer of

---

* 1 kilopascal is approximately equal to 10 centimetres of water.

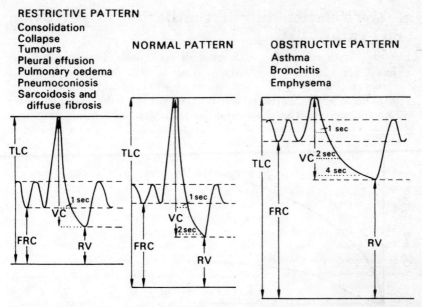

RESTRICTIVE PATTERN
Consolidation
Collapse
Tumours
Pleural effusion
Pulmonary oedema
Pneumoconiosis
Sarcoidosis and
   diffuse fibrosis

NORMAL PATTERN

OBSTRUCTIVE PATTERN
Asthma
Bronchitis
Emphysema

Fig. 1.1. Lung volumes. The divisions of the lung volumes are shown in their normal proportions in the centre and, at the sides, the changes seen in restrictive and obstructive patterns of abnormality.

Vital capacity + Residual volume = Total lung capacity

(VC)   (RV)   (TLC)

carbon monoxide across the lungs (transfer factor, TLco) is reduced. The stiffness of the lungs is described in terms of **compliance**, which is the relation of the change in volume of the lung per unit of pressure required to inflate it. Unfortunately, compliance is difficult to ascertain as it requires measuring the pleural pressure with an oesophageal balloon. Reduction in compliance leads to an increase in the work of ventilation. This extra work may itself consume all the extra oxygen transferred across the lungs as the result of the increased ventilation.

2. Perfusion of the lungs

In normal subjects perfusion of the lungs with blood is not entirely uniform. The lower parts of the lungs receive more blood flow than the upper parts due to the effect of gravity. There is greater unevenness of perfusion in obstructive and other lung diseases. Pulmonary emboli cause obstruction to pulmonary arteries. There is probably some compensation by the lungs for the effects of emboli in that airways in the affected regions also tend to close. However, this compensatory mechanism is not perfect and some areas of the lungs are therefore ventilated but not perfused. Abnormalities of perfusion are not on the whole improved by artificial ventilation.

3. The relationship of ventilation to perfusion (V̇/Q̇ ratio)

The 'ideal' ratio of ventilation (litres of air per minute) to perfusion (litres of blood per minute) in an alveolus is about 0·8. The consequences of disturbance of the V̇/Q̇ ratio are different for oxygen and carbon dioxide. This is because of differences between the shape of the carbon dioxide (CO_2) and oxygen (O_2) dissociation curves which are shown in Fig. 1.2.

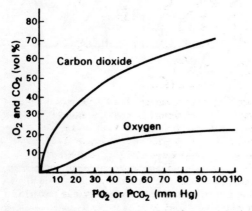

Fig. 1.2. Oxygen and carbon dioxide dissociation curves. (In SI units, 1 kilopascal equals 7·5 mm Hg)

When all the alveoli in the lung are uniformly ventilated and perfused in the ratio of 0·8 then the pulmonary venous blood has a Pco_2 of about 40 mm Hg (5·3 kPa) and a Po_2 of about 100 mm Hg (13·3 kPa). In pulmonary disease, particularly asthma and chronic obstructive lung disease, there is reduction of ventilation to some alveoli so that some are ventilated normally and others ventilated ineffectively as illustrated in Fig. 1.3. In this Figure it is assumed that there is no over-all increase in ventilation: there is therefore a reduction in Po_2 in the underventilated alveoli and hence in the corresponding alveolar capillaries. This leads to a reduced oxygen tension in the pulmonary venous blood and in the systemic arterial blood. Similarly, carbon dioxide is not effectively removed from the underventilated alveoli so that its concentration rises in the pulmonary venous and systemic arterial blood. This rise causes an increased drive to ventilation, the effect of which is to increase over-all ventilation and, in particular, ventilation to those parts of the lung which are open. As the dissociation curve for carbon dioxide (Fig. 1.2) is approximately straight over the relevant part, increased ventilation of some alveoli can compensate for decreased ventilation to other alveoli; this may be enough to restore the Pa_{CO_2} to normal levels.

The situation for oxygen is not so satisfactory and is illustrated in Fig. 1.4. Hyperventilation of the open alveoli increases the Po_2 of the blood leaving those alveoli, but since the oxygen dissociation curve is virtually flat

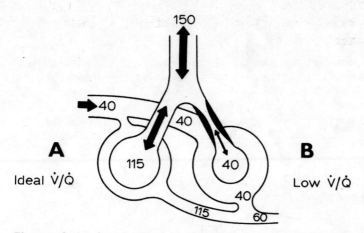

Fig. 1.3. Gas-exchanging lung compartments are represented by the two rounded areas; the branching tubes leading into them depict airways. Surrounding each compartment is a channel representing the capillary network which is supplied by a pulmonary arteriole and which empties into a pulmonary venule. The arrows represent ventilation and perfusion, and their thickness is proportional to the magnitude of ventilation or perfusion. The numerals indicate oxygen tensions in mm Hg at the various sites (divide by 7·5 to obtain kPa).

The ratio of ventilation to perfusion is normal in compartment **A**, but, owing to airway obstruction, ventilation is grossly reduced in proportion to perfusion in compartment **B.** Consequently, the Po_2 of blood leaving this compartment is 40 mm Hg and the Po_2 of the mixed blood leaving both compartments is 60 mm Hg (8 kPa) (normal Po_2, 95 mm Hg or 12·7 kPa).

at a Po_2 above 95 mm Hg (12·7 kPa) (Fig. 1.2) there is only a minimal increase in oxygen saturation of the blood from these alveoli. The mixed pulmonary venous and systemic arterial Po_2 is therefore still low, even when hyperventilation is sufficient to bring the Pa_{CO_2} back to normal.

The above description implies that in the normal subject there is an 'ideal' $\dot{V}/\dot{Q}$ ratio of all alveoli throughout the lung. In practice this is not the case. There appears to be a scatter of $\dot{V}/\dot{Q}$ ratios which have a mean of about 0·8. The less scatter, the more efficient is the over-all ventilation; the greater the scatter, the more inefficient is gas transfer in the lungs. In normal people gravity tends to increase the scatter of $\dot{V}/\dot{Q}$ ratios. There is more blood flow and more ventilation to the alveoli in the dependent parts of the lungs than to the upper parts of the lungs. However, there are bigger top to bottom differences in perfusion than there are in ventilation. In other words, there is much more ventilation in the upper parts of the lungs than there is perfusion ($\dot{V}/\dot{Q}$ ratio as high as 3·0). Conversely, there is relatively less ventilation at the bases of the lungs than there is perfusion ($\dot{V}/\dot{Q}$ ratio as low as 0·6).

These figures apply to normal healthy non-smoking men breathing quietly above functional residual capacity (FRC) in the upright position. When a normal subject expires below his FRC, the small airways start to close off. The lung volume at which these airways close is called the **closing**

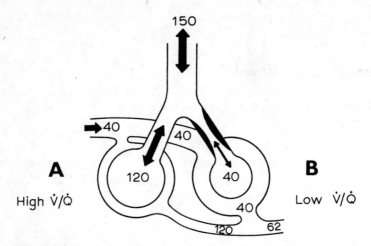

Fig. 1.4. Symbols are the same as for Fig. 1.3. This diagram illustrates that even when ventilation is increased so that some compartments of lung have an abnormally high $\dot{V}/\dot{Q}$ ratio (**A**), these compartments cannot compensate for the impaired oxygen uptake of those with a low $\dot{V}/\dot{Q}$ ratio (**B**), and the Po_2 of the mixed blood leaving both compartments is still only 62 mm Hg (8·3 kPa) (normal Po_2, 95 mm Hg or 12·7 kPa).

volume. Such closure of small airways can be detected in children and in adults but not in adolescents. With increasing age the lung volume at which small airways close off become progressively larger, and between the ages of 50 and 65 (depending on smoking habits) small airways are closing off during quiet tidal breathing; in other words, closing volume is above FRC. When small airways are closed off before the end of normal expiration in this way there is severe reduction of ventilation and of the $\dot{V}/\dot{Q}$ ratios at the bases of the lungs. Smoking, obesity, operation, certain drugs and the supine posture all increase the closing volume and lead to an overall deterioration in respiratory function.

Closure of airways in dependent lung regions, and impairment of $\dot{V}/\dot{Q}$ ratio, is common in patients being ventilated. For this reason it is often advisable to introduce a positive pressure effective at end-expiration, which keeps the lungs from collapsing down to that lung volume at which closure becomes a problem; in other words, effective FRC is increased above closing volume. Between 2 and 10 cm H_2O (0·2–1·0 kPa) **positive end-expiratory pressure** (PEEP) usually serves this purpose.

It helps to understand the concept of the $\dot{V}/\dot{Q}$ ratios if the lung is visualized as a three-compartment model.

1. Part of the lung has alveoli with normal or 'ideal' $\dot{V}/\dot{Q}$ ratios.

2. A second part has very low $\dot{V}/\dot{Q}$ ratios; this can be thought of as a portion of the perfusion failing to reach alveoli and being wasted as though it had passed through an anatomical shunt, i.e. venous admixture.

3. A third part of the lung has a high $\dot{V}/\dot{Q}$ ratio; this can be thought of as a portion of the ventilation failing to reach the alveoli and being wasted

as though it had ventilated only dead space, i.e. increased physiological dead space.

References and bibliography

Bates, D. V., Macklem, P. T. and Christie, R. V. (1971). *Respiratory Function in Disease*, 2nd edn. W. B. Saunders, Philadelphia, Pa., and Eastbourne.

Campbell, E. J. M., Dickinson, C. J. and Slater, J. D. H. (1975). *Clinical Physiology*, 4th edn. Blackwell Scientific, Oxford.

Cherniack, R. I. M., Cherniack, L. and Naimark, A. (1972). *Respiration in Health and Disease*, 2nd edn. W. B. Saunders, Philadelphia, Pa., and Eastbourne.

Comroe, J. H. Jr. (1974). *Physiology of Respiration*, 2nd edn. Year Book Medical Publisher, Chicago.

Cotes, J. E. (1975). *Lung Function*, 3rd edn. Blackwell Scientific, Oxford.

Sykes, M. K. and Vickers, M. D. (1970). *Principles of Measurement for Anaesthetists*. Blackwell Scientific, Oxford.

Chapter 2

Respiratory Failure—Diagnosis and Treatment

Chronic respiratory failure

Extrapulmonary thoracic disease

Chronic respiratory failure may be due to impaired ventilatory function of the chest wall and diaphragm as in obesity, kyphoscoliosis, ankylosing spondylitis and diaphragmatic paralysis.

Chronic restrictive pulmonary disease

Disorders involving a progressive replacement of lung parenchyma by fibrous or other tissue cause a restrictive pattern of lung disorder:

1. Fibrosing alveolitis of unknown aetiology (cryptogenic) or due to inhaled allergens (extrinsic).
2. Diffuse granulomatous conditions, such as sarcoidosis, Wegener's granulomatosis, tuberculosis.
3. Occupational lung disease, such as coal worker's pneumoconiosis, silicosis, asbestosis.
4. Collagen diseases, such as polyarteritis nodosa, disseminated lupus erythematosus.

The predominant symptom of restrictive lung diseases is shortness of breath, particularly on exercise. Sufferers are frequently little disturbed at rest and often sleep well, even when lying flat. On examination, they can be cyanosed and sometimes show finger clubbing. Crackles are heard with the help of a stethoscope over the affected areas of lung. Lung function testing reveals a restrictive pattern (see page 2).

Other chronic lung diseases can lead eventually to respiratory failure, but may have commoner presentations in the initial stages. An example is bronchiectasis, which may cause sputum and cough for many years and only when the disease is very extensive does it lead to respiratory failure.

Chronic obstructive pulmonary disease

In clinical practice we are more usually concerned with the problem of chronic obstructive lung disease which is by far the commonest cause of respiratory failure in Britain. In these patients lung function testing reveals an obstructive pattern (see pages 2, 29).

Two types of chronic respiratory failure are distinguishable: in one there is hypoxaemia without hypercapnia; in the other there is hypoxaemia with hypercapnia. The signs and symptoms depend on which of these conditions is predominant.

Hypoxaemia alone

In patients with intact compensatory mechanisms, hyperventilation is enough to maintain normal levels of Pa_{CO_2}, even when the disease is far advanced. However, as already explained in the section on the $\dot{V}/\dot{Q}$ ratios (see page 4), the level of hyperventilation sufficient to reduce the Pco_2 to normal frequently does not restore the Po_2 to normal in diseased lungs. Such patients, with chronic obstructive lung disease and a normal Pa_{CO_2} but reduced Pa_{O_2}, have been graphically described as 'pink puffers'. Their history is more of increasing shortness of breath than of cough and sputum. Clinically they tend to be thin and are often barrel chested. Although hypoxaemic, this is often not sufficiently severe to cause central cyanosis at rest, and peripheral circulation tends to be good so that there is no additional peripheral cyanosis. Hyperventilation at rest is usually conspicuous and on exercise becomes extreme. The hypoxaemia is exaggerated on exercise and may develop into frank cyanosis. Pink puffers usually show few or no signs of right-sided heart failure and on chest x-ray the heart is of normal size but there is usually radiological evidence of emphysema.

Sometimes, emphysema presents in young people whose only symptom is increasing shortness of breath; in a few of these there is an inherited deficiency of a_1 antitrypsin which normally inhibits the excessive destruction of lung tissue by the enzyme, trypsin.

Hypoxaemia with hypercapnia

In this type of respiratory failure there is a low Pa_{O_2} combined with a raised Pa_{CO_2}. These patients, like pink puffers, have severe abnormalities of $\dot{V}/\dot{Q}$ ratios, but there is insufficient increase in ventilation to compensate for the rise in Pa_{CO_2} caused by the $\dot{V}/\dot{Q}$ disturbance. The reasons for the failure of the respiratory system to respond to the rise in Pa_{CO_2} are not clear. At one time it was thought that such patients were those whose disease had simply become more severe than those with hypoxia alone, but this is unlikely as patients can die with hypoxaemia without ever developing a rise in Pa_{CO_2}. These patients may have some inherent reduction in sensitivity of the respiratory system to the rise in Pa_{CO_2}. Alternatively, it may be that the disease itself imposes some malfunction on the central nervous system. Such patients have been well described as 'blue bloaters'. They have usually been cigarette smokers and have had a persistent cough with sputum for years. They tend to be obese and are not markedly short of breath at rest. They have some central cyanosis and, usually, conspicuous peripheral cyanosis. They frequently develop right-sided heart failure, indicated by raised jugular venous pressure, peripheral oedema and an enlarged tender liver. Chest x-ray usually shows some cardiac enlargement but not emphysema. The electrocardiograph frequently shows evidence of right ventricular hypertrophy.

Patients with hypercapnic respiratory failure frequently have an increase in blood volume and in red cell mass as a physiological reaction to hypoxaemia. Sometimes this polycythaemia is out of proportion to the level of hypoxaemia and may in itself cause problems due to the increased viscosity of the blood.

It should be emphasized that the two types of patient described above are at the extreme ends of a clinical spectrum of chronic obstructive lung disease. In practice many patients have some of the features of both types and cannot be clearly placed in one or other category. Probably the most useful distinguishing feature is the level of Pa_{CO_2} as this has important therapeutic consequences (see oxygen therapy, page 19).

Acute respiratory failure

Acute respiratory failure may be caused by:

1. Impairment of ventilation by acute disorders of the nervous system, chest wall, diaphragm or pleura.
2. Obstruction of the larynx or trachea.
3. Acute disorder of the lung parenchyma; i.e. pneumonia, adult respiratory distress syndrome, idiopathic distress syndrome in the newborn.
4. Obstructive airways disease.
5. Anaesthesia and surgical operation.
6. Heart failure.
7. Pulmonary embolism.

1. Impaired ventilation

Central nervous system

Drugs are the commonest cause of central nervous system depression of ventilation. Self-administered overdose of hypnotics such as opiates, barbiturates, diazepines or other hypnotics is increasingly frequent. Depression of respiration may also follow the therapeutic administration of drugs for the control of pain, anxiety, mania or indeed following anaesthesia for operative procedures. Brain injury following, for example, severe trauma or hypoxic damage can cause respiratory failure. Any central nervous disease sufficiently severe to cause coma can also cause ventilatory failure and among these are meningitis, encephalitis, diabetic coma, hypothyroidism, brain stem or other cerebrovascular accidents and raised intracranial pressure.

Peripheral nervous disorders

Poliomyelitis involving the phrenic nerve nucleus in the cervical cord used to be a common cause of respiratory failure. Now rare in Europe, it still occurs in other countries. Patients with myasthenia gravis or the myasthenic syndrome, which is associated with carcinoma, may develop acute ventilatory failure. It is particularly likely to occur after thymectomy for myasthenia gravis. Peripheral neuropathies may be sufficiently severe to affect the intercostal or phrenic nerves. This can occur in the Guillain–Barré syndrome, or the polyneuritis associated with carcinomas. Drugs such as nitrofuratoin can cause peripheral neuropathies, as can the ingestion of poisons such as the heavy metals, particularly lead. The phrenic nerve can be paralysed due to invasion by carcinoma and occasionally as a result of infections. Paralysis of one hemidiaphragm may tip a patient over into respiratory failure.

Muscle disorders

Muscles may be paralysed following the use of muscle relaxant drugs during anaesthesia or on other occasions. Some subjects are slow to excrete these drugs and may need artificial ventilation whilst neuromuscular conduction is restored. Streptomycin and neomycin potentiate the action of the non-depolarizing relaxant drugs such as tubocurarine and result in prolonged apnoea. The myopathies may eventually affect the respiratory muscles.

Rib cage disorders

Multiple rib fractures may produce an area of the chest wall that is functionally separate from the rest of the thoracic cage. This flail segment may move paradoxically inwards on inspiration and thus impede ventilation. If the flail segment is sufficiently large, respiratory failure may ensue.

Acute disorders of the pleura

Pneumothorax

Pneumothorax, whether spontaneous or secondary to some investigative procedure such as needle biopsy of the lung, results in chest pain and shortness of breath. When the leak in the pleura allows air to enter during inspiration or during coughing, but does not allow it to leave during expiration, increasing dyspnoea occurs as the intrapleural pressure rises resulting in compression of the lung and mediastinal displacement (tension pneumothorax). The patient becomes progressively more short of breath and cyanosed and may lose consciousness and die unless the pressure in the pleural space is relieved. In an emergency this is simply done by pushing any available wide-bore needle through an intercostal space in the axilla. The air whistles out and the patient rapidly recovers. More definite treatment requires an indwelling intercostal catheter leading to an underwater seal.

Acute collection of fluid in the pleural space

Fluid in the pleural space may prove on sampling by aspiration to be straw-coloured serous fluid, blood or even chyle. When such fluid collects rapidly, progressive shortness of breath occurs. Emergency treatment is to aspirate the fluid and, if possible, deal with the cause.

2. Obstruction of the larynx or trachea

Croup syndrome

The upper airways in children are small and more easily obstructed than in adults. Clinically the important sign is inspiratory stridor. There is severe dyspnoea with central cyanosis, marked use of the accessory muscles of inspiration and indrawing of the supraclavicular fossae and lower costal margins on inspiration. This syndrome may be due to the following:

Diphtheria

Obstruction of the larynx by diphtheritic membrane is a disease of the past in Europe but still occurs elsewhere and may require tracheostomy.

Acute obstructive laryngo-tracheo-bronchitis

This is most commonly due to viral infection, sometimes with bacterial superinfection by streptococci or staphylococci. In addition to dyspnoea and inspiratory stridor, there is fever and hoarseness or actual aphonia. If treatment with antibiotics for the possible bacterial superinfection and steam inhalations is not successful, intubation and ultimately tracheostomy may be required.

Epiglottitic and supraglottic oedema

This is usually due to *Haemophilus influenzae* type B infection. The clinical features are similar to acute obstructive laryngotracheal bronchitis except that there is no voice change as the larynx is not involved. Antibiotic treatment with ampicillin and cloxacillin or gentamicin and lincomycin should be started without hesitation. Tracheostomy may become necessary.

Acute laryngeal oedema

Angioneurotic oedema due to acute hypersensitivity to a drug, bee sting, shell-fish or other protein may cause life-threatening acute laryngeal oedema requiring emergency tracheostomy.

Acute laryngeal oedema may complicate prolonged tracheal intubation.

Inhaled noxious gases may cause pulmonary oedema with or without laryngeal involvement.

Inhaled foreign body

Children put an assortment of foreign bodies in their mouths for exploratory purposes and sometimes inhale them. Adults are more likely to inhale foreign bodies such as teeth when they are unconscious as a result of alcoholic intoxication or during anaesthesia for dental extractions or operations on the mouth or for bronchoscopy.

Healthy adults can inhale food when they talk and eat at the same time; the incidence is greater in women than men. A piece of meat impacted in the larynx causes acute airway obstruction. Children should be turned upside down but this is not a practical proposition in adults. Adults are treated by the Heimlich manoeuvre which can be life saving. The operator puts his arms round the patient from behind with one hand over the other fist over the xiphisternum. A sharp jerking movement up under the sternum may dislodge the food, otherwise emergency laryngotomy on the dining room floor may be necessary!

3. Acute disorders of lung parenchyma

Pneumonia

Pneumonia is a common cause of respiratory failure, particularly in young children, debilitated adults and the elderly. It is commonly due to bacteria, but may be caused by viruses, mycoplasma or other organisms. Treatment is with appropriate antibiotics, oxygen and physiotherapy. Despite these measures, artificial ventilation is sometimes necessary.

Idiopathic respiratory distress syndrome in the newborn (IRDS)

IRDS was formally known as hyaline membrane disease. It occurs in premature babies whose immature lungs lack surfactant. Parts of the lungs are therefore unable to expand and the premature infant develops central cyanosis with tachypnoea, expiratory grunting and sternal retraction, usually within four hours of birth. If the infant survives, fibrin exudes into the alveoli and forms a fibrinous matrix which enmeshes protein material and forms the hyaline membrane lining the alveoli.

As a result of the anoxaemia there is a metabolic acidosis which is further compounded by the raised Pa_{CO_2} due to the ventilatory failure. This acidaemia completes the vicious circle by causing a rise in pulmonary vascular resistance and further depresses the amount of oxygen taken up by blood traversing the lung.

Treatment is highly specialized and should only be undertaken in a specialist neonatal care unit. It aims to maintain the vital functions until enough surfactant forms.

Attention must be given to maintenance of temperature, acid–base status, and humidity and oxygen concentration of inspired air. Too much oxygen (for instance, a Pa_{O_2} above 120 mm Hg or 16 kPa) carries the danger of retrolental fibroplasia.

Constant positive airway pressure (CPAP) techniques apply a constant inflating pressure of 6–12 mm Hg (0·8–1·6 kPa) to the lungs of the spontaneously breathing neonate. Various methods of achieving this have been suggested but it is difficult to obtain in a spontaneously breathing neonate. If it is not effective or if there are frequent apnoeic periods, artificial ventilation becomes necessary.

Adult respiratory distress syndrome

There are a group of disorders which all present similarly, as follows:

1. Abrupt onset of dyspnoea.
2. Widespread râles on auscultation.
2. Marked hypoxaemia and cyanosis.
4. Chest x-ray shows widespread dense fluffy shadowing similar to that of gross pulmonary oedema. Because of their similar presentation and because it is often difficult to establish the exact cause, these conditions have been grouped together and called the adult respiratory distress syndrome (ARDS).

Some causes of adult respiratory distress syndrome are:

Shock lung
Near-drowning
Fat embolism
Multiple pulmonary embolism
Acute viral pneumonia
Inhalation of acid vomit
Certain adverse drug reactions, e.g. heroin and methadone overdose
Acute pancreatitis
Inhalation of noxious gases, e.g. smoke
High altitute pulmonary oedema

Of these causes of adult respiratory distress syndrome, some merit further description.

Shock lung

Shock lung may occur in patients who have suffered several traumas or systemic shock. It may follow massive operations and particularly cardiopulmonary bypass, severe sepsis, major non-thoracic trauma, prolonged ventilation and other severe systemic upsets. In the past it was known as 'congestive atelectasis'. The presentation is of 'wet lungs' due to pulmonary oedema without evidence of cardiac failure. There is hypoxia due to disturbed V/Q ratio with resulting hyperventilation and hypocapnia until the terminal stage, when hyperventilation is insufficient and the Pa_{CO_2} starts to rise.

Pathology. At autopsy, patients dying of shock lung show a whole spectrum of abnormalities representing not only the presumed specific lesions but also those of complicating factors such as bronchopneumonia.

The specific lesions are believed to be thromboemboli in the small pulmonary vessels. There is interstitial and intra-alveolar oedema and often hyaline membrane formation. There is evidence of increased capillary permeability and loss of lung surfactant resulting in areas of atelectasis. There are petechial haemorrhages on the pleura and focal areas of congestion as well as atelectasis within the lung substance.

Mechanism. A great deal of experimental work has been done on the mechanism of shock lung. The important suggested mechanisms can be summarized as follows:

1. The lungs readily become overloaded by transfused fluids. Non-colloids distribute in extravascular tissues and cause pulmonary oedema without elevation of central venous pressure.

2. Lung surfactant is diminished or lost as a result of damage to type II alveolar cells which normally produce it.

3. Microembolism of the pulmonary capillaries occurs as a result of intravascular coagulation due to the shock itself and also as a result of transfusion of stored blood.

4. Acidosis and hypoxia cause arterial vasoconstriction, an increase in pressure in the postcapillary venules and increased capillary permeability resulting in patchy areas of congestion.

Clinically. Four phases are described:

Phase I	Period of shock.
	Spontaneous hyperventilation and hypocapnia.
Phase II	Early respiratory distress.
	Hypoxia due to shunting of 10–20% cardiac output.
	Hyperventilation and hypocapnia.
Phase III	Gross hypoxia: mechanical ventilation required.
	Chest x-rays show 'shock lung'.
Phase IV	Terminal anoxaemia with final carbon dioxide retention.

Treatment. Apart from treatment of the shock itself with prompt restoration of blood volume, patients should initially be given a high concentration of oxygen by mask. If the Pa_{O_2} cannot thus be maintained over 70 mm Hg (9·3 kPa) or the Pa_{CO_2} starts to rise, artificial ventilation should be begun. These patients have stiff lungs with low lung volumes and a low FRC because of the amount of unventilated lung.

Additional measures that have been advocated are:

1. Intravenous cyproheptadine (Periactin) to discourage platelet aggregation and for its antiserotonin effect.

2. Heparin by continuous infusion unless contraindicated.

3. Low molecular weight dextrans to reduce platelet aggregation.

4. Diuretics for pulmonary oedema.

5. Corticosteroids may be helpful in shock lung. It is customary to give methylprednisolone 1–4 g daily by injection, though objective evidence of benefit is lacking.

Inhaled acid vomit

Vomiting does not occur in patients properly prepared for anaesthesia but may occur in the course of emergencies and particularly during labour. Inhalation of acid vomit may cause a severe haemorrhagic pneumonia (Mendelson's syndrome). There is delayed onset of fever with dyspnoea and cyanosis; sometimes there is wheezing; the chest x-ray shows widespread diffuse shadowing as in the other forms of acute respiratory distress syndrome. Treatment is by pulmonary lavage and systemic corticosteroids and antibiotics.

Near-drowning

Inhalation of fresh or salt water can result in near-drowning, with a patient who may be unconscious, apnoeic and even pulseless. Emergency treatment is to clear the airway and start artificial ventilation with cardiac massage if there is no pulse. Even if apparent recovery occurs, all victims of near-drowning with aspiration must be admitted to hospital because the irritation of the alveoli by the inhaled water can result in later pulmonary oedema, the syndrome of 'secondary drowning'. This pulmonary oedema of secondary drowning may require artificial ventilation.

4. Acute obstructive airways disease

Bronchial asthma

Asthma is characterized by intermittent episodes of bronchoconstriction. Sometimes these may be merely irritating but occasionally they can be life threatening. Known asthmatics who present with an exacerbation of symptoms should be taken seriously: the patient is usually a good judge of his disability. On examination he is dyspnoeic, usually wheezy and sometimes frankly cyanosed. Auscultation characteristically reveals widespread wheezes, but occasionally there is so little movement of air that the chest may be virtually silent. This represents very severe status asthmaticus and should be treated accordingly. A chest x-ray should be taken to rule out pneumothorax, pneumonia or other causes of the dyspnoea.

Treatment

Aminophylline is given as a slow bolus of 250 mg intravenously followed by 500 mg 6-hourly in a 5% dextrose drip. Salbutamol is an excellent alternative which has recently become available as an intravenous infusion.

Although such bronchodilators may reduce obstruction they may initially cause a paradoxical fall in Pa_{O_2} due to redistribution of blood flow; 40% oxygen should be given by an MC or similar mask. Skilled physiotherapy may help clear retained secretions, especially if it is preceded by a bronchodilator such as salbutamol given by the Bird respirator at the bedside. Hydrocortisone 200 mg is given intravenously initially and this dose repeated hourly until a response is obtained. Prednisone 40–60 mg daily should be started orally.

Anaphylactic shock

Anaphylactic shock usually follows within seconds or minutes of the injection of a drug to which the patient has previously become sensitized. The patient is apprehensive and restless; there may be sneezing, running nose, facial oedema, urticarial rash and itching. There may be tightness in the chest and a feeling of suffocation with bronchospasm and pulmonary oedema. Peripheral circulatory collapse can follow. Initial treatment is with subcutaneous adrenaline (1 ml of 1 : 1 000 sol.) intravenous hydrocortisone (200 mg) and intramuscular chlorpheniramine (10 mg).

Acute exacerbation of chronic bronchitis

Patients suffering from chronic airways obstruction are often precipitated into respiratory failure and unconsciousness when given potent analgesics, particularly morphine and pethidine, for the treatment of pain due to an injury or to myocardial infarction. Patients with kyphoscoliosis are similarly very susceptible to the effects of narcotics.

Patients with chronic airways obstruction may develop a pneumothorax with dyspnoea but without much pain. This can cause a sudden deterioration in their ventilatory capacity. This remediable condition may be dismissed as an exacerbation of chronic respiratory failure unless an erect chest x-ray is taken.

Patients with normal lungs may develop respiratory failure if they sustain enough rib fractures but patients with chronic obstructive airways disease are precipitated into respiratory failure by much less severe chest trauma. The pain of even one fractured rib—and they can be fractured by coughing—can inhibit a patient's cough so that the retained secretions cause sublobar and even lobar collapse. If, in addition, narcotic drugs are given to control the pain, respiratory failure may readily occur. In these patients the pain should be controlled by local anaesthetic blocks.

Patients with chronic airways obstruction develop exacerbations which may be due to viral or bacterial infections, exposure to dust, fumes, fog or smoke, and may occur, particularly in the winter, for no obvious reason.

Clinical assessment

During an acute episode these patients present with a severe exacerbation of their symptoms and in particular with severe shortness of breath.

It is important to measure the blood gases and electrolytes. Measurement of the pH gives an indication of how long the Pa_{CO_2} has been raised. When this has been elevated for some time the kidney retains bicarbonate and the pH is approximately normal whereas in acute respiratory failure there is not time for such buffering and the pH is low; it may be as low as 7·2.

Routine measurements of haemoglobin, total and differential white blood count, serum electrolytes and urea should be performed. Chest x-ray and ECG should be taken and some simple assessment of respiratory function such as the PEFR made.

Treatment

Whilst the role of bacteria in exacerbations is not always obvious, patients with an acute exacerbation of chronic obstructive lung disease should be treated with broad spectrum antibiotics, such as amoxycillin, co-trimoxazole or oxytetracycline. If there has been an exacerbation of right heart failure, diuretic therapy should be instituted or increased. Frequently there is an increase in bronchial obstruction and this may be relived with bronchodilators. Oral prednisone should be given in severe cases if it is thought that there is bronchoconstriction. Venesection is occasionally beneficial in patients who have a gross increase in haemoglobin and circulating red cell mass, but objective evidence for its efficacy is largely lacking.

Physiotherapy

It is helpful to give saline or a bronchodilator such as salbutamol by assisted positive pressure ventilation with the Bird ventilator and follow this by physiotherapy to help the patient cough up sputum.

Sedation

It is very dangerous to give any sedative drugs, including such apparently mild ones as the phenothiazines and other tranquillizers even in small doses, to patients with chronic respiratory failure as they can cause severe and sometimes fatal respiratory depression. There is a particular danger when these patients are admitted to hospitals where it is usual practice to prescribe night sedation for all patients. In those patients with respiratory failure this may be a prescription for death.

Respiratory stimulants

A drug which stimulated the respiratory centre and increased ventilation would be of great value in the treatment of respiratory failure. A number of drugs such as nikethamide, amiphenazole, vanillic acid diethylamide, prethcamide and dimefline have been advocated as respiratory stimulants. Most of these do appear to act as general central nervous system stimulants and temporarily improve ventilation a little. However, the advantages are small and in effective dosages they produce convulsions and hypomania so that few of them are ever used in British practice. The newest respiratory stimulant is doxapram, which is claimed to have an improved action and fewer side effects.

Oxygen therapy (see chapter 6, p. 41)

Hypoxaemia affects myocardial and cerebral function. Below a Pa_{O_2} level of 30 mm Hg (4 kPa) it may cause coma and death. It is therefore logical to try to raise Pa_{O_2} by oxygen therapy but this has certain dangers and should only be given in known concentrations with certain precautions.

The most satisfactory way of giving known concentrations of oxygen is by the disposable Ventimask. There are four types, delivering 24%, 28%, 35% and 40% oxygen respectively. The principle of the masks is that a jet of oxygen draws a standardized flow of air through holes at the base of the mask by the venturi effect. It is therefore important that these holes should not be obstructed by tape, tubing or the like.

The key to safe oxygen therapy is measurement of the arterial blood gases. If the Pa_{O_2} is greater than about 50 mm Hg (6·7 kPa), there is probably no need for added oxygen in the absence of complications. Below this level the patient is on the steep part of the oxygen dissociation curve (see Fig. 1.2) and oxygen therapy should be considered.

In patients in whom the Pa_{CO_2} is normal, an increase in inspired oxygen may greatly relieve symptoms. Oxygen should be administered by a Ventimask giving 35% or 40% inspired oxygen. If there is any deterioration in the patient's level of consciousness, the blood-gas estimates should be repeated. If the Pa_{CO_2} has risen then the level of inspired oxygen should be reduced by using a Ventimask giving only 24% inspired oxygen.

Dangers with oxygen therapy arise in patients in whom the Pa_{CO_2} is raised or in whom the Pa_{CO_2} is not known because it has not been measured. These patients may be made worse by giving oxygen. This is because patients with chronic hypercapnic respiratory failure depend for their respiratory drive not upon pH or Pco_2 in their arterial blood, but upon anoxic stimulation of the aortic and carotid chemoreceptors. Thus if the anoxia is relieved by oxygen therapy the respiratory drive is lost, leading to hypopnoea or apnoea and a consequent further rise in Pa_{CO_2}. Pa_{CO_2} may rise to 80, 100 or even 120 mm Hg (10·7, 13·3 or 16 kPa) and at these levels causes coma and even death. Unfortunately, the clinical signs of carbon dioxide intoxication are so similar to those of the underlying respiratory failure that the situation is frequently not recognized. The most useful clinical indication of worsening hypercapnia is deterioration in the mental state through confusion to coma. Sometimes the administration of oxygen results in such a rapid loss of consciousness that it is too fast to be accounted for by just a fall in ventilation; it is thought that this may be due to a sudden reduction in the carbon dioxide carrying capacity of the blood consequent upon its higher oxygen saturation. This leads to unloading of carbon dioxide and an abrupt increase in mixed venous and arterial Pco_2.

In patients with carbon dioxide retention, oxygen should therefore be given initially in low concentrations (24%) and the arterial blood gases measured again. The concentration of oxygen in the inspired air can be increased to 28% provided progress is satisfactory. If the Pco_2 rises in spite of such judicious oxygen therapy, artificial ventilation must be considered.

5. Post-operative respiratory failure

Following operations, patients may develop respiratory failure due to shock lung (p. 14) or due to mechanical factors.

Anaesthetics and drugs given during the anaesthesia and for postoperative analgesia tend to cause depression of the respiratory and cough centres. Respiratory movements are also diminished by pain, particularly following abdominal or thoracic surgery. Dried secretions tend to be retained after anaesthesia and this may cause atelectasis. Patients often lie supine after operations, which may cause a reduction of FRC below the level of closing volume, thus allowing parts of the lung to close during tidal breathing; sublobar and lobar collapse may follow.

Some of these factors cannot be avoided after operations but patients should be encouraged to move and cough frequently; they should be treated with vigorous physiotherapy.

Giving routine antibiotics postoperatively is probably ineffective and encourages the development of antibiotic-resistant bacteria in the patient and the hospital.

6. Left ventricular failure secondary to cardiovascular disease

Severe pulmonary oedema causes respiratory failure. This may follow damage to the left ventricle due to myocardial infarction, cardiomyopathy or other causes. Alternatively, it may be due to fluid overload following extensive blood or other fluid transfusion or to inefficient excretion of fluid as in renal failure. Treatment of left ventricular failure and fluid overload is to give a powerful short-acting diuretic such as frusemide 40–80 mg intravenously, repeated if necessary. Oxygen should be given in high concentration. A 40% Ventimask or an MC mask are suitable. Morphine (10 mg i.v. or i.m.) or diamorphine (5–10 mg i.v. or i.m.) tend to reduce pulmonary oedema. The blood volume can be reduced by venesection of 500 ml of blood; an alternative is to apply sphygmomanometer cuffs to the limbs to restrict venous return and reduce the overload on the right ventricle.

7. Pulmonary embolism

Pulmonary embolism can present in many clinical guises. One of them is respiratory failure with unexplained dyspnoea, hyperventilation and even with wheezing. Another may be recurrent attacks of pain and shortness of breath with progressive deterioration of lung function. There may be right-sided heart failure due to the rise in pulmonary artery pressure and the ECG may show right heart strain. The chest x-ray usually shows shadows due to areas of pulmonary infarction but may show underperfusion of lung areas. A lung scan may then reveal filling defects.

Treatment is initially with continuous intravenous heparin maintained until there is clinical improvement. Then oral anticoagulant therapy with warfarin is continued, usually for several months.

Bibliography

Campbell, E. J. M. (1960). A method of controlled oxygen administration which reduces the risk of carbon dioxide retention. *Lancet*, **2**, 12.

Crofton, J. and Douglas, A. (1975). *Respiratory Diseases*. Blackwell Scientific, Oxford.

Drug and Therapeutics Bulletin (1976). Idiopathic respiratory distress syndrome in the newborn. **14**, 37.

Wardle, E. M. (1974). Post traumatic respiratory insufficiency: what is 'shock lung'?. *J. Roy. Coll. Physns. Lond.* **8**, 251.

Chapter 3

Indications for Tracheostomy and Laryngotomy

Tracheostomy has been practised for many years to overcome obstruction of the upper respiratory passages. In the past it was used most frequently in the treatment of patients dying with diphtheritic or streptococcal membranes occluding their pharynx or larynx. The serious debility that was associated with the membrane formation often made the patient's death likely in spite of the tracheostomy. As a result, tracheostomy acquired a sinister reputation and was considered only as a desperate last resort. In more recent years, with the success of the prophylactic treatment for diphtheria, tracheostomy was frequently performed to prevent the aspiration of food and pharyngeal secretions into the trachea in patients with disordered swallowing reflexes, often as the result of bulbar poliomyelitis or head injury. It was also used to overcome the airway obstruction produced by malignant disease or by trauma of the pharynx and larynx or following laryngectomy. Until 1950, these were the main indications for tracheostomy. The operation was never lightly undertaken and apart from its use in laryngectomy it was seldom a planned procedure.

Between 1950 and 1967, the operation of tracheostomy was performed with increasing frequency. In the United Oxford Hospitals only 18 tracheostomies were performed in 1950; in 1959 there were 76 (McClelland, 1965). The reason for this enormous increase in the number of tracheostomies performed at that time was that the indications were widened to make it part of the treatment of various types of ventilatory failure and to forestall possible respiratory obstruction in cases of facial trauma and injury to the neck. Since 1967, prolonged tracheal intubation, especially by the nasal route, has been increasingly practised. Tracheostomy is now carried out less frequently as initial treatment in patients needing artificial ventilation (see Chapter 16). When a tracheostomy is to be performed it should be a planned procedure and not a desperate bedside emergency. Institution of an early tracheostomy or endotracheal intubation may allow further ventilatory deterioration to be forestalled.

Tracheostomy carries a small morbidity and mortality as it bypasses the protective mechanisms operative in the nose and pharynx; it also lessens the patient's ability to cough effectively. As a result, it may be justified to give more conservative methods of treatment a trial so that the advantages to be gained may be weighed against the risks. In these cases it is usual to temporize using an endotracheal tube inserted either through the mouth or through the nose.

Endotracheal intubation and tracheostomy

Until recently any patient who was to be ventilated for longer than 48 hours underwent tracheostomy. Though there is general agreement that rubber endotracheal tubes should not be left in place for longer than 24 hours, the development of cuffed plastic tubes which are less irritant to the larynx and trachea has increased interest in prolonged intubation.

This technique has many advantages. Intubation is an everyday procedure and may be performed repeatedly on the same patient. Many of the complications of tracheostomy, both immediate and late, are avoided and the absence of any surgical incision means there is no permanent scar.

However, fixation of the tube is more difficult and, because of its greater length, aspiration of secretions may be less successful. If the tube is too short the cuff may damage the larynx, and if too long there is risk of ulceration of the carina and of bronchial intubation. Many patients do not tolerate an endotracheal tube without heavy sedation and this may delay the return to spontaneous respiration.

Nasotracheal intubation seems to cause less discomfort than oral intubation. Unless there is a definite contraindication, it is probably the route of choice as less sedation is required and oral toilet can be carried out more easily. However, it does have certain disadvantages. The additional length of tube may make the aspiration of secretions more difficult, and trauma to the nose, nasal septum and nasopharynx are not uncommon. The tube may pass behind the nasal mucosa into the retropharyngeal space as it is being introduced, and ulceration of the septum and alar cartilages has been reported.

There is no agreed time limit to prolonged intubation, though if ventilation has to be continued, it is usual to perform a tracheostomy after a maximum of 7–10 days. If it is probable that at least 2 weeks' artificial ventilation will be necessary or that the return to spontaneous respiration may be difficult and prolonged, there are undoubted advantages to an early tracheostomy.

Laryngotomy

Occasionally a desperate situation arises with alarming rapidity; for example, following aspiration of a foreign body, trauma to the larynx or in an acute infective condition—especially laryngotracheitis in infants. Under these compelling circumstances the operation of tracheostomy is difficult and too time consuming. The difficulty arises from the excessive respiratory effort being made by the patient which causes excessive movement of the neck muscles, the distended veins that may accompany coughing as the patient tries to clear his airway and the hypertension consequent upon hypoxia and hypercarbia, and the agitated state of the patient. In these circumstances laryngotomy quickly establishes an airway, relieves the patient's hypoxia and anxiety, and allows a route through which an anaesthetic can be administered for a definitive planned tracheostomy operation. In situations where an emergency tracheostomy may be required, one must decide whether the risk to the patient is sufficient to perform the operation prophylactically; if not, a knife suitable to perform laryngotomy and a tube to act as an airway should be immediately available.

The indications for tracheostomy and laryngotomy may be summarized under the following headings:

1. To overcome airway obstruction above the level of the stoma.
2. To separate the pharynx from the larynx and so prevent aspiration of secretions and food.
3. To allow the mechanical aspiration of secretions from the tracheo-bronchial tree.
4. To allow prolonged artificial ventilation.
5. As part of certain planned procedures on the head, neck and larynx.

1. To overcome airway obstruction above the level of the tracheostome

This can occur at various levels in the upper air passages from the mouth and tongue down to the larynx and upper trachea. The causes may be either congenital or acquired, the result of trauma, inflammation or new growth. Trauma and new growths are probably the commonest causes of this form of obstruction. Severe facial injuries involving the mandible and floor of the mouth may necessitate a tracheostomy before reparative surgery can be undertaken. Infective lesions of the soft tissues of the floor of the mouth, causing Ludwig's angina, and extensive operations upon the lower jaw, can produce respiratory obstruction due to the associated oedema and bruising. Occasionally, respiratory obstruction results from radiation therapy to laryngeal tumours. Bleeding into a thyroid cyst may necessitate urgent tracheostomy or laryngotomy. Sometimes a similar situation will result from an allergic response as a part of the syndrome of angioneurotic oedema, producing oedema of the soft tissues and respiratory obstruction. This may develop with alarming suddenness. Respiratory obstruction occasionally occurs as the result of nervous lesions. Bilateral abductor palsy of the vocal cords following recurrent laryngeal nerve damage, airway obstruction by an uncontrollable tongue following bilateral hypoglossal nerve trauma or serious swelling of the tongue, will cause respiratory obstruction. This may result from injury to the tongue or the nerve supply or from lesions of the brain stem. An uncuffed tracheostomy tube usually suffices to maintain an airway in these conditions; however, the inability to swallow saliva is an indication for the use of a cuffed tube.

2. To separate the larynx from the pharynx

If the swallowing reflex is disturbed or if the contents of the pharynx are likely to overwhelm the patient's laryngeal reflexes, tracheostomy should be performed. The swallowing reflex involves sensory input from the posterior third of the tongue and the posterior pharyngeal wall by means of the glossopharyngeal nerve to initiate the reflex. In order that fluid and food be successfully swallowed, in all but trained individuals, the tongue must project the food back into the oropharynx and on to the posterior pharyngeal wall. During swallowing the larynx is elevated; this, together with narrowing of the laryngeal orifice, effectively deflects food into the oesophagus and prevents aspiration into the trachea. Disturbances of this reflex can occur from sensory loss, loss of central reflex control, from interference with the innervation of the muscles concerned or due to interference with mechanical integrity of the swallowing act. It is often possible to temporize by nursing the patient on his side or in the head-down position or by inserting a cuffed nasotracheal tube into the trachea, but a tracheostomy should be performed if the disease process makes it likely that the duration of the disorder will be prolonged. Head injury, bulbar palsy, glossopharyngeal nerve palsy, pseudo-bulbar palsy, surgical interference with the sensitive posterior pharyngeal wall and posterior third of the tongue and deep coma may depress the patient's swallowing and laryngeal reflexes. In these circumstances it is usually necessary to use a cuffed tracheostomy tube to protect the larynx from the contents of the pharynx.

3. To allow the aspiration of tracheobronchial secretions

If the secretions of the tracheobronchial tree are unusually copious or tenacious, or the patient's powers of expectoration are reduced, it may be necessary to perform a tracheostomy in order to allow mechanical aspiration of the secretions and so prevent the patient from drowning in his own secretions. Simpler measures, such as nursing the patient in an atmosphere of high humidity combined with postural coughing, may be tried initially. If this fails and the accumulated secretions collect in the lungs, then segmental or lobar collapse of the lung may occur. This may cause shunting of venous blood through unventilated areas of lung and cause arterial hypoxaemia. This inevitably weakens the patient still further and lessens his ability to cough effectively.

The sputum produced by laryngo-tracheo-bronchitis in small children and neonates is often so tenacious that these feeble children find it impossible to clear it from their tracheobronchial tree. The small diameter of their air passages and the relative ineffectiveness of their cough makes this a hazard to their life. In these children, tracheostomy, humidification of the inspired air and efficient suction of their secretions can be life saving. In recent years nasotracheal intubation has been tried with success in the treatment of this condition to avoid the necessity for tracheostomy. By this means difficulties of decannulation are obviated in these children. In adult patients a combination of a depressed cough reflex and excessive tenacious sputum may result in the inability to expectorate tracheobronchial secretions. This is seen postoperatively and during debilitating illnesses. The coughing power of the patient may be depressed by mechanical disabilities such as results from poliomyelitis, fractured ribs, obesity, upper abdominal incisions, nasogastric tubes and when brochospasm occurs. It may also be the result of depression of the brain by excessive doses of drugs, especially in the postoperative period. The disadvantages of tracheostomy in these patients are relatively small and the benefits to be gained considerable. There is therefore little reason for not considering tracheostomy early in these patients. An uncuffed tube should be used whenever possible in the treatment of these conditions as it is safer should a plug of sputum block the tracheostomy tube. If this occurs, the patient will still be able to breathe around the tube. An uncuffed tube also has the advantage of causing less hindrance to the actual mechanism of coughing.

4. To allow prolonged artificial ventilation

Prolonged artificial ventilation through a cuffed endotracheal tube presents difficulties and dangers that can be reduced if a tracheostomy tube is used as the airway. The long length of the endotracheal tube together with its relatively narrow bore makes it difficult to keep clean and free of inspissated secretions. The resistance to the flow of gases along such a tube may result in a prolongation of the passive expiratory phase unless a negative subatmospheric phase is used to assist exhalation. Deaths have occurred in patients receiving artificial ventilation as a result of the endotracheal tube becoming twisted or kinked in some part, causing undue resistance to ventilation (Robbie and Feldman, 1963). The use of a non-kinking flexometallic tube lessens this danger.

It is generally recommended that, unless there is some contraindication, a tracheostomy should be considered after 3–4 days of intubation, and endotracheal intubation should not be continued for more than 10 days except in special situations, as permanent damage to the vocal cords may otherwise result. In any event, an endotracheal tube should be changed every 24–48 hours. If the patient is making such progress that he may be expected to be breathing adequately on his own within the next few hours, or his condition suggests that he is beyond hope of recovery, then it may be decided to continue ventilation through the endotracheal tube. In neonates and small children, tracheostomy carries special problems (Chapter 13). In these circumstances it may be preferred to continue artificial ventilation through a nasotracheal tube as long as this is considered safe.

5. As part of a planned procedure on the head, neck or pharynx

Major surgery involving extensive and multi-stage procedures upon the mandible, pharynx and larynx may require a tracheostomy to allow the safe administration of anaesthesia and to obviate the risk of postoperative oedema or haematoma accumulating in the tissues of the neck, causing respiratory obstruction. Many of these patients present difficult intubation problems for the anaesthetist, especially if there is ankylosis or malformation of the jaw or if there is a friable haemorrhagic tumour of the pharynx or larynx. In these patients a preoperative tracheostomy under local anaesthesia might be considered advisable. If the larynx is to be removed surgically a permanent, end-opening tracheostome will be required.

References

McClelland, R. M. A. (1965). Complications of tracheostomy. *Brit. med. J.*, **2**, 567.

Robbie, D. S. and Feldman, S. A. (1963). Experience with fifty patients treated by artificial ventilation. *Brit. J. Anaesth.*, **35**, 771.

Chapter 4

Indications for Artificial Ventilation

Assessment of the severity of respiratory failure

Clinical observations

It is often possible to decide just from looking at a patient that he is in severe respiratory failure and needs artificial ventilation. Unconsciousness or impending coma indicate severe failure. Short of unconsciousness, a patient may look and be exhausted by the sheer mechanical work of breathing. He may be unable to talk at rest or to cough. Gilston (1976) has described some of the common facial signs that indicate respiratory distress, such as open mouth panting which may occur despite the presence of a tracheostomy, 'clicking of the tongue' which is often associated with a 'jaw tug', tightening and pursing of the lips (this has an effect similar to positive end-expiratory pressure (PEEP)), flaring of the ala nasae, prominent contraction of the sternal part of the sternomastoid muscle and sweating of the forehead. All or any of these signs may draw attention to the need for artificial ventilation.

Hypoxaemia may be detected by looking for central cyanosis in the mucous membranes of the lower lip and tongue. This sign is subjective and difficult, particularly in artificial light. The blue colouration is due to the quantity of unsaturated haemoglobin in the glood and is therefore more difficult to assess when the patient is anaemic. Central cyanosis becomes recognizable when arterial saturation is 80% or less ($Pa_{CO_2} \leqslant 50$ mm Hg or $\leqslant 6.7$ kPa). There can therefore be severe reduction of Pa_{O_2} without clinical cyanosis. By the time cyanosis can be recognized, the Pa_{O_2} has reached the steep part of the oxygen dissociation curve (see Fig. 1.2) and further small reductions in Pa_{O_2} cause large falls in saturation. Below a Pa_{O_2} of about 40 mm Hg (5.3 kPa) central nervous symptoms of hypoxia such as tiredness, headache and loss of judgement are found. Patients with an arterial Pa_{O_2} of 25 mm Hg (3.3 kPa) are likely to be comatose, and an arterial Pa_{O_2} of 20 mm Hg (2.7 kPa) is probably the lowest compatible with survival. Peripheral cyanosis as seen in the hands and feet is a sign of poor peripheral circulation or decreased perfusion at the periphery and may or may not be associated with central cyanosis. A blue colouration may also be seen in methaemoglobinaemia and sulphhaemoglobinaemia, but this is not improved when additional inspired oxygen is given.

Hypercapnia is more difficult to recognize. The first signs are muscle twitching and coarse tremor. At higher levels of Pa_{CO_2} there may be headache, confusion, impairment of consciousness and eventually coma. Papilloedema due to raised intracranial pressure is described but very rarely seen in practice.

Simple lung function testing

The degree of ventilatory impairment and its progression can be assessed by some simple tests of ventilatory function such as FET, PEFR, $FEV_{1.0}$ and VC (Table 4.1).

TABLE 4.1.   NORMAL VALUES FOR SOME LUNG FUNCTION TESTS

Test	Abbreviation	Units (SI units)	Range*
Forced expiratory time	FET	sec (s)	< 4·5
Peak expiratory flow rate	PEFR	l/min (l min⁻¹)	300–600
Forced expiratory volume in one second	FEV_1	litres (l)	1·5–4·0
Forced vital capacity	FVC	litres (l)	2·0–5·5
$FEV_1/FVC \times 100$		%	65–85
Residual volume	RV	litres (l)	1·0–2·5
Functional residual capacity	FRC	litres (l)	2·0–5·0
Total lung capacity	TLC	litres (l)	3·0–8·0
RV/TLC ratio		%	25–40
Airway resistance	Res.	cm H_2O/l/sec (kPa l⁻¹ s⁻¹)	< 2·0 (< 0·2)
Transfer factor (for carbon monoxide)	TLco	ml/cm H_2O/min (mmol kPa⁻¹ min⁻¹)	18–40 (6–13)
Compliance	CL	ml/cm H_2O (l kPa⁻¹)	100–300 (1·0–3·0)

* Normal values depend on sex, age and height; for tables relating these variables see Cotes (1975).

Tidal volume and minute ventilation may be measured at the bedside with a Wright respirometer (see Fig. 11.1). The respirometer is usually used to measure ventilation over 1 or 2 minutes. To obtain tidal volume the minute volume is divided by the respiratory rate. Measurements may be compared with the predicted normal values obtained from Radford's nomogram (Fig. 4.1).

Arterial blood-gas measurements

The clinical signs of hypoxaemia and hypercapnia, as described above, are subjective and variable and the only effective way of determining the overall efficacy of respiration is by measuring the arterial blood gases. Unfortunately, this is still considered a major procedure in many hospitals and the technique is not as widely available as it should be.

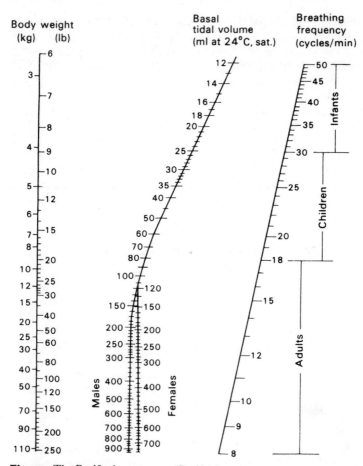

Fig. 4.1. The Radford nomogram (Radford et al., 1954, *N. Engl. J. Med.*, **251**, 878). By plotting a straight line between body weight and the breathing frequency required, a basal tidal volume may be predicted. Remember this tidal volume must be increased in hyperpyrexia and artificial ventilation (increased dead space). Corrections to be applied to predicted basal tidal volume:

Daily activity (i.e. patients not in coma): add 10%
Fever: add 9% for each degree above 37° C (rectal)
Altitude: add 8% for each 1 000 m above sea level
Tracheostomy/endotracheal tube: subtract 1 ml/kg body weight
Metabolic acidosis during anaesthesia: add 20%
Dead space of anaesthesia apparatus: add volume of apparatus and mask dead
  space.

Arterial blood should be taken into a freely moving 5 or 10 ml syringe via a standard venesection needle. The syringe should be lubricated with heparin and a small amount left to fill the dead space. Usually the easiest site for sampling is the femoral artery but the radial and brachial arteries are also widely used by the more experienced. The skin overlying the artery is infiltrated with local anaesthetic. About 5–10 ml of blood should be taken, avoiding contamination by air. Any small air bubbles that do collect should be expressed immediately and the syringe capped. The puncture site should be pressed firmly for at least 3 minutes. The blood sample should, if possible, be analysed immediately or, if not, should be stored in ice for not more than 4 hours before analysis.

Capillary blood samples taken from the lobe of the ear may be used as a substitute for arterial gas samples but in the clinical situation this method is less reliable.

Alveolar and hence mixed venous carbon dioxide tension can be measured by the rebreathing technique of Campbell and Howell (1962). Arterial carbon dioxide tension is estimated as 6 mm Hg (0·8 kPa) greater than this. This method is less reliable than blood gas estimations and has the disadvantage that it does not give information as to Pa_{O_2} or pH.

Indications for artificial ventilation

General

The large number of different conditions which may lead to respiratory failure have been described above. Some indication of how these should be treated initially have been given. If such treatment is not successful then respiratory function may deteriorate to the extent that artificial ventilation must be considered.

Artificial ventilation is an undignified and uncomfortable procedure for patients and, even in the best managed units, exposes them to a greatly increased risk of lung infections, particularly with gram-negative bacilli. Artificial ventilation should not be undertaken in patients who are dying of irrecoverable diseases, as for example, the end stages of motor neurone disease or lymphangitis carcinomatosa. On the other hand, it is clearly obligatory in diseases which are likely to improve with time, such as asthma, flail chest, poisoning or acute infective polyneuritis. In some situations the choice may depend on both clinical and moral judgement, as for example in pneumonia of the elderly, exacerbations of chronic bronchitis and apparently irreparable brain damage. Under these circumstances it is difficult to give more than general guidance. If there is a chance that the patient may return after the illness to a reasonable existence then artificial ventilation may be worthwhile. On the other hand, if the progress of the disease is inexorable it seems meddlesome to maintain life for days or weeks merely for its own sake. It is much harder to stop ventilation when the patient is clearly not going to recover than not to start in the first place.

Artificial ventilation needs to be carried out in a carefully controlled intensive care environment and is expensive in resources and the time of doctors, nurses and ancillary staff. The problems and difficulties of managing these patients require special training and organization. If suitable facilities are not available locally, it is better to transfer the patient before the need for ventilation has become urgent, or disasters have occurred during ventilation.

Indications in specific conditions

Central nervous system disorders

In the majority of intensive care units in general hospitals throughout the United Kingdom, the largest single aetiological factor in necessitating artificial ventilation is self-induced poisoning. In these patients confusion and coma may occur before respiratory failure. This may also occur in encephalitis, meningitis and other central nervous system disorders. Patients who are unconscious because of drugs or in the postoperative period cannot be tested for vital capacity or peak flow rates as it necessitates co-operation. In these patients blood gases must be the indicator for artificial ventilation which should be considered if there is an otherwise unexplained fall in Pa_{O_2} of over 20 mm Hg (2·7 kPa) or rise in Pa_{CO_2} to 50 mm Hg (6·7 kPa).

Ventilation is frequently necessary following severe brain trauma and hypoxic episodes such as occur during diabetic coma or epileptic fits. In patients with brain damage it is extremely difficult to predict the likely prognosis and these patients should be given the benefit of any doubt and should receive artificial ventilation when significant changes in blood gases are detected. It is especially important to prevent any rise in carbon dioxide tension in these patients as it will be associated with an increase in intracranial pressure and will prejudice the cerebral circulation. It is therefore usually advisable to start artificial ventilation in these patients if the Pa_{CO_2} is elevated above 45 mm Hg (6 kPa).

Peripheral nervous disorders

Most of these disorders are potentially reversible. Respiratory function in these patients can deteriorate alarmingly without revealing any obvious signs on clinical examination. It is important to measure frequently the vital capacity in patients with poliomyelitis, infective and other polyneuritis and acute myasthenia. A rapid reduction of vital capacity to one-half predicted value or an acute fall to less than 1 litre in an adult are indications for ventilation. Even at these levels of vital capacity such patients may have only mild hypoxia, but it is dangerous to delay active ventilation until gross hypoxia or carbon dioxide retention occurs. Such changes may herald the rapid onset of serious deterioration with the possibility of cardiac arrest. It is better to ventilate too early than too late. Patients with myasthenia gravis who become refractory to treatment with neostigmine, or who have a myasthenic crisis or who have ACTH therapy often benefit from a period of artificial ventilation during which time they need not receive neostigmine therapy and the sensitivity to the drug is usually restored.

Disseminated sclerosis is a disease in which intermittent exacerbations occur but which sometimes improves with time. It is therefore reasonable to treat an acute episode of respiratory failure with artificial ventilation.

Muscle disorders

Tetanus and the prolonged effects of muscle relaxants are potentially reversible and if they cause respiratory failure must be treated with artificial ventilation. The muscle disorders such as the myopathies and motor neurone disease are progressive and irreversible and are not an indication for ventilation unless there has been an acute superadded problem such as pneumonia. Even then it may be unkind to ventilate such a patient as death is likely to come soon in spite of temporary relief.

Disorders of the thoracic cage

Injury to the thoracic cage following trauma or thoracic operations may require artificial ventilation due to the mechanical defect. However, care must be taken not to overlook some remediable cause, such as a pneumothorax, before embarking upon artificial ventilation in these patients. The need for artificial ventilation may be assessed by measuring the vital capacity. It is not usually necessary or desirable to wait for hypoxia before ventilating patients with severe thoracic mechanical difficulties. On the other hand, kyphosis and ankylosing spondylitis are chronic long-standing conditions and such patients should not usually be ventilated even if they develop carbon dioxide retention. It may occasionally be necessary to ventilate them during an episode of respiratory failure due to some acute cause such as may occur during the recovery period following an operation.

Pulmonary indications

Chronic obstructive lung disease. It has been realized increasingly that the treatment of chronic obstructive lung disease with artificial ventilation in itself tends to cause further damage to the lungs and such patients are often difficult to wean from the ventilator. The only indication is an acute exacerbation which appears to be reversible and the patient seems likely to be left with good enough respiratory function for a reasonable existence thereafter. If, for example, a patient with chronic obstructive lung disease is inadvertently given inappropriate night sedation, a short period of artificial ventilation while the drug is being excreted may allow him to return to his previous state.

Chronic restrictive lung disease. It is not usually useful to treat these patients with artificial ventilation unless there has been an acute episode in addition to the chronic restrictive lung disease and the life style following the illness is likely to be acceptable.

Occasionally the restrictive lung condition is the temporary result of surgical interference such as may follow the repair of a large ventral hernia, when the increased intra-abdominal pressure prevents the normal descent of the diaphragm. Artificial ventilation is often indicated following repair of large diaphragmatic hernias, especially in neonates.

Acute pulmonary disease. Acute lung diseases should be treated conservatively in the first instance as described in Chapter 2. If this fails, artificial ventilation may become necessary. A rise in Pa_{CO_2} above 50 mm Hg (6·7 kPa) in a subject who was previously normal is usually an indication for artificial ventilation. Many patients need artificial ventilation before this stage is reached; this has to be assessed on clinical grounds. In pneumonia, if there is a steady increase in pulse and respiratory rate, increasing general exhaustion and shortness of breath on talking, artificial ventilation should probably be started. If status asthmaticus is not reversed by conservative treatment the patient may become weak and tired and this is the moment to start ventilation, even if there has been no rise in Pa_{CO_2}.

Cardiovascular disorders

If pulmonary oedema due to left ventricular failure cannot be controlled by the usual medical treatment, artificial ventilation should be instituted. Continued production of frothy sputum with severe shortness of breath and worsening hypoxia despite all medical treatment are the indications for ventilation in this situation.

Other causes

There remains a further group of patients in whom the indications for artificial ventilation are less easily quantified. They are the patients recovering from an acute exacerbation of a chronic disease or from the effects of an operation and anaesthesia, in whom the work of respiration appears to be out of proportion to the actual amount of ventilation achieved. Often these patients are able to produce an adequate tidal volume with some effort and their blood gases are maintained at a border line level. These patients are easily exhausted by a bout of coughing, they can only speak a few words at a time and they appear anxious lest their ventilation should fail. In these patients a period of artificial ventilation is often beneficial. It also allows the patient to receive sedatives and analgesics if required, without the risk of precipitating respiratory failure.

References

Campbell, E. J. M. and Howell, J. B. L. (1962). Rebreathing method for measurement of mixed venous P_{CO_2}. *Brit. med. J.*, **2**, 630.

Cotes, J. A. (1975). *Lung Function*, 3rd edn. Blackwell Scientific, Oxford.

Gilston, A. (1976). Facial signs of respiratory distress after cardiac surgery. *Anaesthesia*, **31**, 385.

Radford, E. P., Ferris, B. G. and Kriete, B. C. (1954). Clinical use of a nomogram to estimate proper ventilation during artificial respiration. *New Engl. J. Med.*, **251**, 877.

Chapter 5

Physiological Effects of Tracheostomy and Artificial Ventilation

Normal physiology

When a patient breathes in there is a co-ordinated contraction of the diaphragm, the intercostal muscles and of the small muscles fixing the larynx to the mandible. This results from an integrated nervous discharge from the hind brain along the phrenic, intercostal and cranial nerves. As inspiration continues, stretch receptors in these muscles and also in the abdominal wall discharge and feed back inhibitory stimuli to the brain, resulting in a cessation of inspiratory effort. Passive exhalation occurs as the result of the unopposed elastic recoil of the lung. Forced inspiration involves contraction of the sternomastoid, scalenus anterior and other neck muscles, whilst forced expiration results from the increase in intra-abdominal pressure caused by the contraction of the abdominal muscles. This helps to raise the diaphragm and expel air from the chest. This is especially important in the presence of increased airways resistance.

During inspiration the glottic opening is at its widest so as to allow the unimpaired passage of air into the chest. As a result of inspiratory effort, the normal elastic resistance of the lung and chest wall is overcome and the lung expands, sucking air into the larynx and trachea, and the intrapleural pressure falls and becomes more subatmospheric than at rest. The oesophagus and other lax intrathoracic organs, such as the great veins, are also affected by this 'sucking force', causing blood to move into the thorax from the abdomen along a pressure gradient. The presence of a functional gastro-oesophageal valve prevents stomach contents from entering the oesophagus, unless the negative pressure developed in the pleural cavity becomes excessive, as may occur when a patient inspires against an obstructed airway.

Abnormal co-ordination of respiration results from depression of the respiratory centres of the brain by drugs, anoxia, trauma and acidaemia. It is also seen in premature and immature babies. It manifests itself as gasping respiration associated with a jerky depression of the chin during inspiration; this has been termed 'tracheal tug'. Tracheal tug results from a failure to fix the larynx during inspiration and is caused by the pull on the trachea, by the lungs, as the diaphragm descends during inspiration. Thus with every contraction of the diaphragm there is a jerky downward movement of the trachea and lower jaw.

The air that enters both lungs is usually inspired through the nose where it is partially warmed and filtered of any large particles. In its passage through the upper airways the air is warmed to body temperature and humidified; saturated air will contain 44 mg of water per litre at 37°C. The drier the inspired air the greater the loss of water from the body during respiration. Also, since the evaporation of water in the airways requires energy, this process will result in cooling of the trachea and bronchial mucosa. Breathing dry cold air therefore results in a loss of fluid and heat by the body.

Effects of tracheostomy

Besides the obvious effect of preventing the patient speaking by circumventing the larynx, a tracheostomy prevents the normal process of warming and humidifying the inspired air. This will produce failure of ciliary activity in the bronchial mucosa, and the normal metachromal ciliary rhythm, by which particulate matter is swept out of the pulmonary tree, will be disturbed. Mucous secretion by the trachea is reduced and it becomes tenacious. Ultimately, squamous metaplasia of the tracheal epithelium occurs.

A tracheostomy bypasses the larynx and upper respiratory air passages, and thereby reduces the resistance to air flow, especially if a pathological process has caused a narrowing of the glottic opening. The reduction in the work of ventilation in patients who have been labouring against progressive narrowing of the air passages produces immediate relief, often in spite of little change in blood gases, as the limitation of ventilation resulting from laryngeal obstruction causes a feeling of impending suffocation in the patient. If the obstruction is of a temporary nature, a similar though less effective reduction of the work involved in ventilatory exchange may be achieved by administering an oxygen-helium mixture to the patient. Because of the lower density of this gas mixture, breathing requires less mechanical effort, allowing a greater gaseous exchange to take place for the same energy expenditure. A tracheostomy reduces the normal anatomical dead space by up to 100 ml; this may be of importance to patients who have a limited tidal volume as it increases the effective alveolar ventilation produced at a given tidal ventilation.

Recently it has become appreciated that a tracheostomy may interfere with the normal elevation of the larynx that takes place in swallowing. This is especially true if an anterior flap tracheostomy has been performed. The patient may be reluctant to swallow, and choking and aspiration of saliva may occur. If the tracheostomy tube is a cuffed one, this may result in accumulation of saliva and other aspirated material in the trachea above the cuff. This stagnant pool of secretions readily becomes infected and may cause tracheomalacia and tracheal dilation.

Many of the complications of tracheostomy are due to pressure effects upon the tracheal wall. Even the pressure in the 'low pressure cuff' type of tracheostomy tube, such as the Portex blue line or Lanz, or a similar high volume, low pressure, cuffed tracheostomy tube, can affect the tracheal mucosa. Pressure effects on the mucosa are likely to be most dangerous during periods of hypotension, tracheal or pulmonary infection and if the patient is receiving steroid therapy. In order that the lateral pressure on the tracheal wall should be kept to a minimum, large lax cuffs are preferred and these should be inflated with just sufficient air to maintain an airtight seal. It should be remembered that the air contained in a cuff will expand as it warms up to the body temperature.

In view of the potential dangers of cuffed tracheostomy tubes, an uncuffed silver tube or a plain plastic tube should be used whenever possible.

Effects of artificial ventilation

As a result of administering IPPV the normal pressure changes in the thorax are reversed. Inspiration now becomes associated with the application of a positive pressure through the airway and lungs whilst exhalation is passive unless a negative phase is used to assist exhalation. The mean intrathoracic pressure is therefore reversed; instead of being a negative value, 4–5 cm H_2O (0·4–0·5 kPa) subatmospheric, as in spontaneous ventilation, it is now positive. As a result of this positive pressure, the pleura, oesophagus and great veins are compressed during inspiration. This will result in intermittently obstructing the blood flow into the chest from the abdomen, unless the pressure in the abdominal veins is greater than that reached in the thorax. Similarly, the passage of blood through the pulmonary circulation will be intermittently impeded if the intrathoracic pressure exceeds the pulmonary artery pressure (normally 18–20 mm Hg (2·4–2·7 kPa) systolic, 8 mm Hg (1·1 kPa) diastolic at the level of the hilum of the lung).

As a result of this increase in intrathoracic pressure, and the concomitant decrease in pulmonary blood flow, there will be a relative overventilation of the lung—areas of the lung will therefore have an increase in V/Q ratio (ventilation–perfusion ratio) and an increase in physiological dead space.

The physiological effects of alterations in the intrathoracic pressure depend upon the efficacy of the body's compensatory mechanisms. These are:

1. Redistribution of the blood so that the venous return is increased.

2. Increase in venomotor tone to raise the venous pressure in the abdomen and so promote venous return against the positive intrathoracic pressure.

3. An increase in alveolar ventilation to compensate for the increase in physiological dead space, caused by the fall in alveolar perfusion that is associated with the increased intrathoracic pressure.

The patient's ability to promote venous return in response to an increase in intrathoracic pressure depends upon the circulating volume and the integrity of the vasomotor centre. Patients who are hypovolaemic as a result of either fluid or blood loss and those whose vasomotor control is depressed by drugs, head injury or spinal cord transection and disease (i.e. acute stages of poliomyelitis) often cannot adjust to these changes. This results in a fall in venous return to the heart and the cardiac output is diminished. This fall in cardiac output may produce both pulmonary and systemic hypotension. However, it has been demonstrated that the majority of patients with an intact circulatory system can readily adapt to the change from subatmospheric to positive intrathoracic pressure and even the positive pressure associated with PEEP does not adversely affect their venous return. Evidence of the increase in venomotor tone in patients on PEEP may often be noted by observing the venoconstriction of the superficial vessels of the hand.

Two other effects of long-term IPPV have been reported. One is a progressive decrease in pulmonary compliance, suggesting a stiffening of the lung tissue. This may be associated with fluid retention in the pulmonary tissue, a form of pulmonary interstitial oedema. Some workers have ascribed this to the effect of flooding the lungs with a high concentration of water particles and blame it upon faulty humidification. The other effect of IPPV that has been described is the occurrence of progressive areas of atelectasis. The atelectasis may be of such a small dimension as to be invisible on an x-ray, but is detected by a progressive increase in the alveolar–arterial Po_2 difference. An increase in this difference suggests that blood is passing through alveoli that are receiving insufficient ventilation. Considerable doubt has been thrown upon the occurrence of progressive atelectasis in the absence of deteriorating pulmonary disease. However, should an increasing A–a O_2 gradient indicate that progressive 'shunting' is occurring, it has been found useful to introduce an end-tidal positive pressure so that the lung is never allowed to deflate to its resting volume. By so doing the alveoli become stabilized and there is less likelihood of spontaneous atelectasis. The other possible explanation for this progressive atelectasis is the suggestion that, as a result of overdistension of the pulmonary alveoli, there may be a diminished secretion of surfactant. Surfactant is secreted by the normal lung alveoli and maintains the integrity of the gas–water interface in the alveoli and prevents the collapse of the alveolar module of the lung. A lack of surfactant will therefore cause alveoli to close more easily and at a larger critical closing volume than would otherwise occur. The suggestion that progressive atelectasis may be prevented by designing ventilators that provide intermittent deep inspiration, the so-called 'artificial sigh', remains unproven.

Effects of abnormal ventilation

By taking away a patient's respiratory control and substituting an artificial ventilatory pattern it is possible either to underventilate the patient or to administer excessive ventilation. Underventilation carries with it the risk of increasing the carbon dioxide tension and unless the inspired atmosphere is enriched with oxygen it will produce progressive hypoxia.

Abnormal ventilation causing hypoxia and hypercarbia or hypocarbia and high oxygen tensions can produce effects upon many organs of the body by affecting basic cellular metabolism, the efficiency with which the haemoglobin carries oxygen from the lungs to tissues and the distribution of blood to various organs. However, in the intensive care unit the effect that probably causes most concern is that upon the cerebral circulation. It has long been known that there exists a regulating system within the cerebral vasculature, in normal areas of the brain, that tends to maintain a normal H^+ ion concentration and CO_2 level of the brain tissue. Any physiological change that would tend to cause a decrease in blood supply, a diminution in oxygen availability or an increase in carbon dioxide tension tends to cause a fall in cerebrovascular resistance and hence an increased blood brain flow. Conversely, hypertension or a raised perfusing pressure, a low Pa_{CO_2} due to hyperventilation and a raised Pa_{O_2}, especially if it is over 500 mm Hg (66·7 kPa), will cause cerebral vasoconstriction. In certain pathological states, such as brain tumours or following a small cerebral haemorrhage, an area of the brain loses this ability to regulate its circulation in response to physiological changes. This effect can be used to encourage these diseased areas to 'steal' blood from normally regulated tissue by deliberately lowering the Pa_{CO_2} by hyperventilation (Robin Hood or 'reverse steal' effect). The compensating effect of a fall in cerebrovascular resistance consequent upon hypotension occurs in animals down to a mean arterial pressure of 40–50 mm Hg; however, hyperventilation at these low pressures may prejudice this normally effective compensatory mechanism. A raised Pa_{CO_2} causes a fall in cerebrovascular resistance and a reduction of the autoregulator effect of hypotension.

The signs of hypoxia include diminution in the level of consciousness, hypertension, tachycardia, restlessness, sweating and nausea; when a significant proportion of the blood is desaturated, cyanosis will occur. It must be appreciated that cyanosis may be a late phenomenon and its recognition is largely subjective; recognition is also dependent upon the type of lighting in the intensive care unit. The only satisfactory safe way of determining whether or not the patient is suffering from hypoxia is to withdraw a sample of arterial blood for analysis of its oxygen content.

Hypercarbia

Hypercarbia produces a release of adrenalin in the body with a resulting hypertension, tachycardia, sweating and tremor. As carbon dioxide accumulation continues, unconsciousness may be produced and at a still later stage cardiac and vasomotor depression will be seen. A diagnosis of hypercarbia can be confirmed either from blood-gas analysis or by analysing the patient's alveolar air.

Hypocarbia

Whilst it is possible that patients will not suffer ill effects from mild degrees of hyper or hypocarbia, the sudden hyperventilation of a patient to a Pco_2 far below his normal will result in restriction of blood flow to the brain and the superficial organs with resulting dizziness, nausea and pallor and coldness of the skin. Gross hyperventilation may result in loss of consciousness. The skin appears cold, cyanotic and vasoconstricted. Hypotension and cardiac arrythmias may occur and renal secretion is diminished.

After a patient has been artificially hyperventilated for a prolonged period, it is likely that his renal compensating mechanisms will have reduced the buffer base of the blood and the CSF in an effort to compensate for the low P_{CO_2}. In these circumstances difficulty may be experienced returning the patient to normal spontaneous ventilation as the patient will have to maintain a high level of alveolar ventilation in order to prevent acidaemia. Extreme hyperventilation to P_{CO_2} below 25 mm Hg (3·3 kPa) may be especially dangerous as it produces EEG changes and evidence of an anaerobic brain metabolism. In patients who are hyperventilated and have not received muscle relaxants or deep central sedation, hyperventilation may produce tetany and carpopedal spasm. This is the result of the changes in ionized calcium and is indicative of changes in the concentration of other partially ionized molecules that may take place. Prolonged hyperventilation to Pa_{CO_2} levels below 35 mm Hg (4·7 kPa) should be avoided except in special situations where it is considered desirable as in localized brain lesions.

Bibliography

Conway, C. M. (1975). Haemodynamic effects of pulmonary ventilation. *Brit. J. Anaesth.*, **47**, 761.

Crawley, B. E. and Cross, D. E. (1975). Tracheal cuffs. A review and dynamic pressure study. *Anaesthesia*, **30**, 4.

Mathias, D. B. and Hedley, J. R. (1974). The effects of cuffed endotracheal tubes on the tracheal wall. *Brit. J. Anaesth.*, **46**, 849.

Chapter 6

Oxygen Therapy—Theory and Practice

Before any discussion can take place on oxygen therapy, certain basic factors concerning oxygen transport need to be grasped.

Oxygen transport

Arterial oxygen **tension** (P_{O_2} in mm Hg or kPa) depends upon adequate breathing (properly called ventilation) and, more important, on the fact that the alveoli of the lung are clear of secretions, are not inflamed and are not collapsed. The latter all increase venous admixture or shunting, thus causing a lowered arterial P_{O_2}. (The arterial oxygen tension is also fundamentally dependent upon an adequate oxygen tension in the inspired gas mixture.)

Arterial oxygen **content** (ml oxygen/100 ml blood) depends largely upon haemoglobin; 1 g of haemoglobin when fully saturated combines with 1·39 ml of oxygen. The way in which oxygen is taken up by haemoglobin (i.e. the relationship between tension and content) is non-linear in the form of an S-shaped saturation curve (Figs. 6.1, 6.2, 6.3 and Table 6.1). The shape

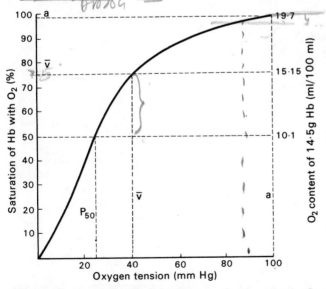

Fig. 6.1. Oxyhaemoglobin saturation curve. On the right the O_2 content of blood of Hb level 14·5 g/100 ml is given. The co-ordinates for arterial blood (a), mixed venous blood (v̄) and also the P_{50} have been added (broken lines).

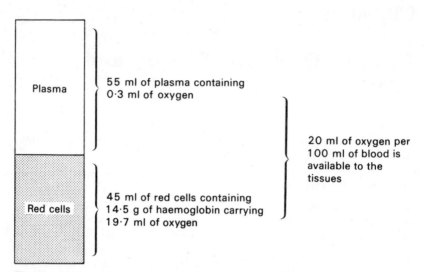

Fig. 6.2. Diagram representing 100 ml of arterial blood of packed cell volume 45% and Hb level of 14·5 g/100 ml, showing the partition of oxygen between red cells and plasma at a Po₂ of 100 mm Hg (13·3 kPa).

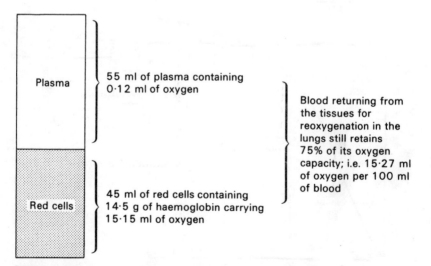

Fig. 6.3. Diagram representing 100 ml of mixed venous blood of packed cell volume 45% and Hb level of 14·5 g/100 ml showing the partition of oxygen between red cells and plasma at a Po₂ of 40 mm Hg (5·3 kPa).

TABLE 6.1.   OXYGEN CONTENT AND SATURATION OF NORMAL BLOOD AT Po_2S VARYING
FROM 10 TO 100 MM HG IN 10 MM INCREMENTS. THE QUANTITIES OF OXYGEN WHICH
DISSOLVE IN PLASMA AT THE SAME Po_2 VALUES ARE ALSO SHOWN

Po_2 (mm Hg*)	O_2 content of 14·5 g of haemoglobin (ml/100 ml)	Saturation of Hb (%)	O_2 content in plasma of 100 ml whole blood (ml/100 ml)
100	19·70	97·5	0·30
90	19·49	96·5	0·27
80	19·09	94·5	0·24
70	18·73	92·7	0·21
60	17·98	89·0	0·18
50	16·87	83·5	0·15
40	15·15	75·0	0·12
30	11·51	57·0	0·09
20	7·07	35·0	0·06
10	2·73	13·5	0·03

*7·5 mm Hg = 1 kPa.

of this curve means that only a very little more oxygen can be carried by arterial blood if the Po_2 is raised above 100 mm Hg (13·3 kPa), and mixed venous blood, with a normal Po_2 of 40 mm Hg (5·3 kPa), is still 75% saturated; i.e. there is a large reserve in the oxygen carrying power of the blood. Even if the Po_2 falls to about 26 mm Hg (3·5 kPa), the haemoglobin is still 50% saturated. (An arterial Po_2 above 50 mm Hg (6·7 kPa) is adequate to support life in a patient provided both mixed venous oxygen and acid–base status are normal, i.e. cardiac output remains adequate.)

The **quantity of oxygen available to any tissue** depends upon the flow of blood through that tissue; e.g. if 100 ml of fully saturated blood flows through the arm in 1 minute then 20 ml of oxygen is available per minute. It follows that the oxygen availability to the **whole body** is equally dependent upon its blood supply, i.e. the **cardiac output**.

Ignoring the amount dissolved in the plasma, the total oxygen availability can be quantified thus:

Oxygen available to the body =
$$1·39 \times Hb \% \times saturation \% \times cardiac\ output$$

Considering some normal values:

$$1·39 \times \frac{14·5}{100} \times \frac{97·5}{100} \times 5\ 000\ ml/minute \rightleftharpoons 1\ 000\ ml/minute$$

The factor 1·39 is a constant, an individual's Hb is constant, and saturation cannot be increased beyond 100%, but cardiac output can be modified from, say, 3 litres per minute during sleep to 25 litres per minute, or more, during exercise. That is to say, the demands for increased tissue oxygenation are met entirely by changes in blood supply or cardiac output.

A different interpretation of the above would be that:

Each   1% change in saturation, when the cardiac output is 5 l/min and the haemoglobin level is normal, accounts for a change of **10 ml/min** in oxygen availability.

Each   1 g change in haemoglobin level, when the cardiac output is 5 l/min and there is full saturation, accounts for a change of **69 ml/min** in oxygen availability.

Each   litre change in cardiac output, when the haemoglobin level is normal and there is full saturation, accounts for a change of **200 ml/min** in oxygen availability

OR the cardiac output is 20 times more important in oxygenating a patient than the actual arterial saturation level.

It follows that measures which raise the cardiac output in low cardiac output shock states (infusion, transfusion and cardiac inotropic drugs, such as isoprenaline, adrenaline and dopamine) are more effective in improving oxygenation than is oxygen therapy by mask, as it is likely that the patient's arterial blood is fully saturated anyway.

Delivery of oxygen to the cells within a tissue depends upon a capillary circulation throughout that tissue; i.e. an **adequate microcirculation**. If a tissue is ischaemic it cannot be oxygenated, no matter what the arterial oxygen content.

Utilization of oxygen within the cells of a tissue depends upon intracellular enzymes.

Forms of hypoxia

It can be seen from the above facts that there exist four basic forms of hypoxia which can ultimately affect tissues.

1. **Anoxic,** where breathing is inadequate or the aveoli are full of exudate, transudate or are collapsed (or where there is a low oxygen tension in inspired gas, e.g. at high altitude).

2. **Anaemic,** where the haemoglobin is low (or when part of the haemoglobin has become combined with something else, such as carbon monoxide from coal gas; or when some of the haemoglobin has become converted to something else, such as sulphaemoglobin or methaemoglobin).

3. **Stagnant,** when tissue perfusion is subnormal for some reason such as cardiac failure, causing increased oxygen extraction from blood and hence venous desaturation.

4. **Histotoxic,** when arterial saturation and tissue perfusion are adequate but the intracellular enzymes have been poisoned, e.g. by cyanide. (This form of hypoxia is obviously of rarity interest only.)

It should be obvious that tissue hypoxia can occur despite a normal arterial saturation because of low flow or cardiac output.

Similarly, normal tissue oxygenation can occur in the presence of arterial desaturation or a low haemoglobin level, because the cardiac output increases.

Tissue oxygenation can be improved by a further adaptive physiological mechanism. An increased haemoglobin production by the bone marrow occurs in man and other animals who reside at high altitudes (low inspired Po_2); in adults with chronic respiratory disease (low arterial Po_2); and, similarly, in children with congenital cyanotic heart disease who often acquire haemoglobin levels above 20 g/100 ml.

Assessment of tissue hypoxia

It should be plain from the facts set out above that the state of oxygenation of a patient's tissues can best be assessed from measurements of **mixed venous oxygen** content. There is one important snag preventing the frequent use of this measurement: mixed venous blood is obtainable only from the pulmonary artery. To obtain a specimen therefore entails the passage of a catheter into a vein and thence via the vena cava and right atrium, through the tricuspid valve to the right ventricle, and through the pulmonary valve into the pulmonary artery. While this can be achieved with Swann and Ganz catheters without too much difficulty, it is a little inconvenient and time consuming for routine clinical application. Recourse is usually made to arterial blood which is easily obtained from a number of sites by simple percutaneous puncture of an artery. Direct measurements of oxygen content are not yet made frequently because apparatus for direct measurement of oxygen tension is more highly developed and gives more easily reproducible (and therefore more accurate) results in unskilled hands. The value obtained has to be applied mentally to the Hb saturation curve for interpretation, especially with regard to changes from previous measurements. (Remember that the difference between 30 and 40 mm Hg (4 and 5·3 kPa) is **18 times** the difference between 90 and 100 mm Hg (12 and 13·3 kPa) in terms of oxygen content—see Fig. 6.1 and Table 6.1.)

Measurement of arterial oxygen tension tells whether the value is normal or not. As they reflect the state of the lungs, serial measurements of arterial oxygen tension tell whether the lungs are getting better or worse under treatment, **provided that one knows the inspired oxygen has not changed from one measurement to the next**.

A measurement of mixed venous oxygen indicates whether the oxygen available to the tissues (arterial content times cardiac output) is adequate to meet the demands of oxygen consumption. As this is not usually measured, the adequacy of tissue perfusion can be inferred from the patient's history and clinical condition and from the measurement of the acid–base status of the arterial blood. If there is a fall in bicarbonate content (i.e. a metabolic acidosis) there is the suggestion that anaerobic metabolism has been or is taking place as a result of tissue hypoxia (provided other causes of metabolic acidosis can be excluded).

Oxygen toxicity

The toxicity of any therapeutic agent should be known before it is applied in an indiscriminate manner. After oxygen had been discovered it was considered that, as it is essential to life, an excess of it would be beneficial to those who are ill. It was also assumed that it had little if any toxic effects.

Oxygen administration, however, may be harmful if arterial oxygen is raised above normal for a particular patient or if the inspired oxygen is higher than 60% at sea level (i.e. in excess of 418 mm Hg or 55·7 kPa). The former can cause and exacerbate respiratory depression and the latter may lead to pulmonary oxygen toxicity (a form of toxic pneumonia).

Respiratory depression

Subjects with chronic respiratory disease (characterized by a permanently raised arterial carbon dioxide tension and a permanently lowered arterial oxygen tension) rely upon their (relative) **hypoxic drive** to stimulate their breathing. When these patients have acute exacerbations of their disease, they pass from relative to absolute hypoxaemia as they slip down the steep portion of their saturation curve. Simultaneously, their arterial carbon dioxide levels rise. Obviously they require oxygen therapy, **but only enough** to push them up to a reasonable oxygen **content**. Too high a Po_2 in their arterial blood would depress their respiration to a degree that would permit carbon dioxide to accumulate, leading to a condition of progressive 'carbon dioxide narcosis' which will cause death if allowed to proceed unchecked.

Only very modest increases in inspired oxygen concentration are adequate to deal safely with these patients; e.g. raising inspired oxygen from 21% (air) to 24% or perhaps 28%.

Oxygen is a very mild respiratory depressant even in normal subjects. In individuals whose respiration is already depressed by drugs (as in self-poisoning cases), indiscriminate elevation of arterial oxygen tension to unnecessarily high levels may have an unfortunate and deleterious effect on ventilation. Oxygen may also depress the vasomotor centre, directly and indirectly, through its effect on the chemoreceptors of the carotid body, causing a fall in blood pressure.

Pulmonary oxygen toxicity

Man is probably the animal who is the least sensitive to the toxic effects of oxygen on lung tissue. In many, pulmonary oxygen toxicity does not develop in less than 24 hours even with an inspired oxygen of 100% and never with an inspired oxygen of less than 50–60% (0·5–0·6 atm. abs.). If higher concentrations than this seem to be necessary in a given clinical situation, then further physiotherapy and artificial ventilation (intermittent positive pressure ventilation—IPPV) via an endotracheal tube or tracheostomy tube may cause a dramatic improvement in oxygenation without the necessity for raising the inspired oxygen. This is due to the beneficial effect of the increase in mean airway pressure in reversing small airways closure and alveolar collapse. The therapeutic benefit of this measure can be furthered under extreme circumstances by raising the pressure in the ventilator during expiration (normally zero, i.e. atmospheric pressure) to which the term 'positive end-expiratory pressure' (PEEP) is applied.

Oxygen therapy

The object of treatment is to increase the oxygen availability to the tissues without giving so much oxygen as to cause toxic effects. Oxygen should be given in such a way that the concentration is known and constant so that the serial measurements of oxygen in blood can be interpreted in terms of improvement or otherwise in lung function (in the case of arterial measurements), or in terms of improvement or otherwise in the relationship between tissue blood flow and oxygen consumption (in the case of mixed venous measurements).

Methods

Oxygen is administered by facemask, nasal catheter and cannula, during the course of artificial ventilation, in a hyperbaric chamber (or bed), by an oxygen tent or by incubator.

Measures increasing oxygen availability

Where appropriate, the following measures must be taken in addition (and sometimes instead of) oxygen therapy.

1. Raise haemoglobin to normal.
2. Increase cardiac output (tissue blood flow) with transfusions, infusions and positive inotropic agents or digitalis as appropriate.
3. Treat the lung pathology as appropriate, i.e. reducing venous admixture and thence improving arterial saturation:
   (a) Physiotherapy.
   (b) Intubation (or bronchoscopy) and suction, or tracheostomy and suction, and IPPV or PEEP.
   (c) Antibiotics as necessary.
   (d) Sometimes steroids (toxic pneumonitis, shock lung, etc.)
   (e) Sometimes bronchodilators.
   (f) Treat congestive cardiac failure with digitalis and diuretics if appropriate.
4. Also measures can be taken to **reduce tissue oxygen demands**:
   (a) Paralysis and IPPV reduce the oxygen cost of breathing.
   (b) Digitalization reduces the oxygen uptake of the heart muscle.
   (c) Prevention of hyperthemia.
   (d) Under extreme circumstances induction of hypothermia by surface cooling to 30° C reduces tissue oxygen requirements by over 50 per cent.

Before considering finally the simple mechanics of giving oxygen via the airway of the patient, one last fact still needs to be appreciated. During inspiration, gas flows into the airways at a peak flow of about 30 l/minute. (As inspiration lasts about 1 second, the inspired volume = 30 000 ml ÷ 60 sec = 500 ml.) Therefore the flow of oxygen mixture given to a patient must be equal to, or in excess of, 30 litres per minute in order that a constant inspired mixture is obtained. When a patient is on a ventilator this objective is achieved. However, most popular oxygen therapy devices used with spontaneously breathing patients supply pure oxygen at a flow rate of much less than this, and the rest of the inspirate is made up by the inspiration of the appropriate amount of fresh air (e.g. MC mask (Fig. 6.4), Edinburgh mask, nasal catheter and nasal cannula).

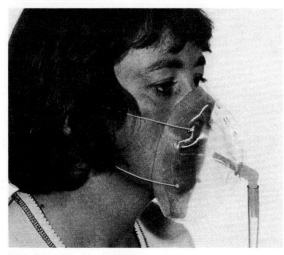

Fig. 6.4. MC oxygen mask

As there is a breath-to-breath variation in peak inspiratory flow rate, this results in a varying amount of fresh air being inspired and hence breath-to-breath variation in inspired oxygen concentration occurs. Furthermore, the average peak inspiratory flow rate varies from subject to subject so that different individuals obtain a different average inspired oxygen concentration even with the same device and the same oxygen flow rate. A further source of variation in inspired oxygen concentration is variation in expiratory pause time (representing oxygen wash-in and carbon dioxide wash-out time), which is more important in the larger capacity devices (these are less popular nowadays; e.g. the Pneumask, Polymask, Oxyaire mask, Portogen mask and BLB mask).

With both the former and the latter groups of devices, the oxygen concentration also varies within each breath as peaks of oxygen of varying degree occur at both the beginning and the end of inspiration.

Yet another source of variation can be produced by variations in fit to the face of the mask from time to time during treatment (i.e. loose or tight fit).

Thus with the devices indicated, it is not possible to know accurately the inspired oxygen concentration at any given moment, and serial measurements of arterial oxygen or, for that matter, of mixed venous oxygen will be robbed of their clinical significance because there is no guarantee that the inspired oxygen has not altered from one measurement to the next. All that the measurements can show under those circumstances is whether the values are normal, but not necessarily whether there is any improvement or deterioration in the patient's condition.

Venturi devices

Fortunately, there are oxygen therapy masks which blow oxygen mixtures at patients in excess of peak inspiratory flow rate, and whose performance is thus independent of patient factors or of fit to the face. These devices operate on the venturi principle (Fig. 6.5) in which pure oxygen entrains a

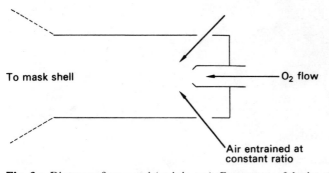

To mask shell

O_2 flow

Air entrained at
constant ratio

Fig. 6.5. Diagram of a venturi (or injector). Emergence of the jet of oxygen causes a zone of negative pressure which entrains a constant ratio of air through orifices in the barrel of the device. The percentage of oxygen obtained remains fixed even though the oxygen flow may vary within limits prescribed by the manufacturer.

constant ratio of room air to produce a fixed concentration mixture. For many years the Ventimasks (Fig. 6.6) have been the only devices available but these have been joined by Mixomasks, Multivents, Accurox and Vario-masks and, no doubt, other masks will follow. There are now available from the various manufacturers devices which give 24%, 28%, 35%, 40%, 50% and 60% oxygen at flow rates in excess of peak inspiratory flow. Their characteristics are:

24% = a ratio of 23 to 1; 2 litres of oxygen entrain 46 litres of air.
28% = a ratio of 10 to 1; 4 litres of oxygen entrain 40 litres of air.
35% = a ratio of 4·4 to 1; 8 litres of oxygen entrain 35 litres of air.
40% = a ratio of 3·1 to 1; 8 litres of oxygen entrain 25 litres of air.
50% = a ratio of 2·5 to 1; ought to be run with a flow of at least 9 litres oxygen entraining 22·5 litres of air.
60% = a ratio of 1 to 1; ought to be run with a flow of at least 15 litres oxygen entraining 15 litres of air.

With these devices, it is possible to give known oxygen concentrations to all spontaneously breathing patients so that any measurements of oxygen, whether in arterial blood or in mixed venous blood, can be interpreted **in the light of a true change within the patient**.

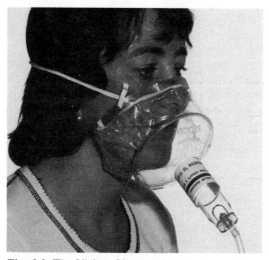

Fig. 6.6. The Vickers Ventimask.

Patients on ventilators

When a patient is on a ventilator an oxygen flowmeter usually delivers oxygen to the machine which pumps a mixture of room air and oxygen to him. Although the resulting inspired oxygen concentration may be constant for long periods, it is not necessarily known. With some modern ventilating systems a chosen oxygen concentration can be selected on a dial so that this problem does not arise.

In the intensive care unit at Guildford the ventilating systems are of the former type and a nomogram is used (Fig. 6.7) in order to obtain oxygen concentration from basic readings of tidal volume, ventilator rate and oxygen flow rate. It is essential in all intensive care practice that inspired oxygen concentration is charted routinely, and certainly that 'blood gases' are always recorded together with the oxygen concentration being administered at the time of blood sampling.

Oxygen tent and incubator

The **oxygen tent** is a device which is now virtually unused in Great Britain for adults. It is of large capacity and fits over a bed so as to enclose a patient's head and trunk. Into the tent, oxygen, which may be humidified and temperature controlled, is blown at a fixed rate. The build-up of oxygen concentration within the tent may take some time. However, since both the tent capacity and the leakage are relatively large, this time may be significantly long. Only the most elaborately constructed oxygen tents are capable of achieving oxygen concentrations in the region of 50%.

Access to the patient is restricted, so that patient care and oxygen therapy may conflict, as the oxygen concentration falls rapidly to that of room air on opening the tent. The risk of fire is greatest with this method.

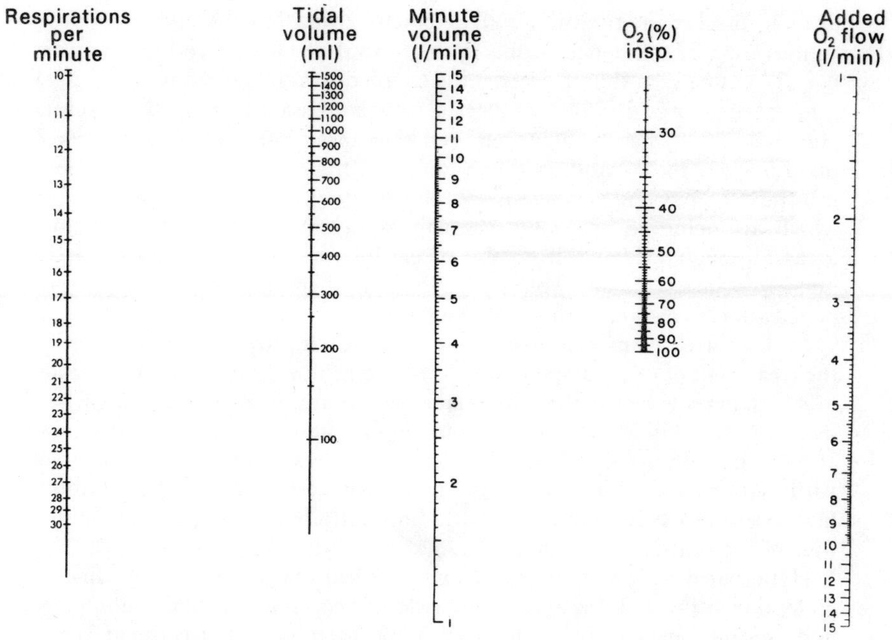

Respirations per minute	Tidal volume (ml)	Minute volume (l/min)	O₂(%) insp.	Added O₂ flow (l/min)

Fig. 6.7. Nomogram used with patients on ventilators for computing minute volumes and mixtures of oxygen in air from minute or tidal volume, respiration rate, and added oxygen flow. The 60% calibration in the oxygen percentage column is printed in red to remind clinicians that it might be better to use PEEP than increase inspired oxygen any further.

The oxygen tent should be reserved for children who are not tolerant of an oxygen mask or nasal catheter. For infants an **incubator** constitutes the only possible method of continuous oxygen therapy and also provides a controlled environment, not only in respect of oxygen concentration, which is normally controlled by a venturi, but also of humidity and temperature. Oxygen concentration build-up is dependent upon the same factors as in the oxygen tent but, because it is a smaller enclosure, it does not take so long to achieve the desired oxygen concentration.

Both the oxygen tent and the incubator, since they enclose the patient entirely, are capable of supplying the mixture at a rate which matches inspiratory flow rate. Unfortunately, as indicated, the concentration may be a varying one.

Hyperbaric oxygen

Reference to the figures given in Table 6.1 with regard to the solution of oxygen in blood plasma, shows that, unlike haemoglobin, the relationship between Po_2 and content in plasma is a linear one although the amount dissolved is very small (at a Po_2 of 100 mm Hg (13·3 kPa) only 0·3 ml of oxygen dissolves in 100 ml blood). Remembering that the normal arterio-venous oxygen difference is only 5 ml/100 ml of blood (see Figs. 6.2 and 6.3), it can be seen that if a patient is exposed to 100% oxygen at about 2½ atmospheres' pressure then an arterial oxygen tension of around 1 700 mm Hg (226·7 kPa) may be achieved, and therefore plasma alone will carry 5 ml of oxygen/100 ml and, in theory anyway, the necessity for haemoglobin transport of oxygen is obviated. Unfortunately, the high capillary Po_2s which are achieved are not necessarily sufficient to oxygenate ischaemic areas although evidence from the successful treatment of arrhythmias in ischaemic heart disease would suggest that there is a slight increase of penetration of oxygen into the damaged tissue.

In short, treatment with hyperbaric oxygen has proved disappointing for the treatment of tissue anoxia and its use seems now to be only worth while in gas gangrene (to combat the anaerobic organisms involved), in carbon monoxide poisoning and in sulphaemoglobin and methaemoglobinaemia. It also may be used in peripheral vascular disease, for the treatment of various ischaemic skin lesions and in chronic osteomyelitis. In addition, high pressure oxygen increases the radiosensitivity of some tumours and is thus of use during radiotherapy for malignant diseases.

Hyperbaric oxygenation may cause cerebral oxygen toxicity leading to epileptiform fits and, because of the risks of occurrence of both pulmonary and central nervous system toxicity, hyperbaric oxygen treatment is not usually given for more than 2 hours at a time, interspersed with rest periods of 1 hour.

References

The following publications by the author have been freely referred to:

(1970). Variation in performance of oxygen therapy devices. *Anaesthesia*, **25**, 210.

(1973). Present practice and current trends in oxygen therapy. *Anaesthesia*, **28**, 164.

(1973). Towards the rational employment of 'the dephlogisticated air described by Priestley'—a study of variation in performance of oxygen therapy devices. *Ann. roy. Coll. Surg. Engl.*, **52**, 234.

(1974). Ideas and anomalies in the evolution of modern oxygen therapy. *Anaesthesia*, **29**, 335.

(1974). Oxygen therapy at ambient pressure. In: *Scientific Foundations of Anaesthesia*, 2nd edn., p. 253. Ed. by C. F. Scurr and S. A. Feldman. Heinemann Medical, London.

(1975). Post-operative oxygen administration. *Brit. J. Anaesth.*, **47**, 108.

Chapter 7

Technique of Tracheostomy

Introduction

Tracheostomy has been described many times over the past two thousand years, though infrequently performed until the nineteenth century (Davison, 1965). The emergency situation demanded the technique of laryngotomy rather than a formal tracheostomy and was inevitably performed for upper airway obstruction, with the dramatic relief of symptoms provided that the bleeding was staunched.

Today there are few, if any, indications for laryngotomy. Most practising physicians are capable of intubating the patient in the emergency situation and then carrying out a tracheostomy later under more controlled circumstances. If, however, intubation proves impossible, a small cannula or needle can be inserted through the cricothyroid membrane and oxygen introduced at a flow of 2–4 l/min. This insufflation technique (Lee and Atkinson, 1973) will give a few minutes for more expert help to become available. Under these circumstances the $P_{A_{CO_2}}$ rises at about 1 mm Hg/min (0·13 kPa/min) while oxygenation remains satisfactory if the lower airway is patent and not obstructed by retained secretions.

Elective tracheostomy

Elective tracheostomy is best performed under general anaesthesia in the operating theatre. Tracheostomy is never performed without good reason, as a result the patient presenting for this operation may have difficulty with breathing and marked airway obstruction. Both these symptoms can produce a mentally distressed patient.

When a tracheostomy is to be performed:

1. the patient should be anaesthetized or adequately sedated
2. the patient should be intubated
3. an intravenous infusion should be set up

Control of the airway and, if necessary, ventilation should be attained before the procedure is begun.

Indications for the use of local analgesia techniques are restricted to the situation where intubation is impossible or where induction is dangerous and intubation uncertain (i.e. where general anaesthesia brings dangers without advantage). Infiltration with local anaesthetic drugs for other reasons is unnecessary.

Preoperative chest and neck x-ray

If there is time, a preoperative chest and neck x-ray can provide valuable information about the size, site and shape of the airway. For example, the upper trachea may be displaced from the mid-line by infection, oedema or tumours of the neck, while the lower trachea, carina and bronchi may be displaced by many pathological conditions in the thorax (Fig. 7.1).

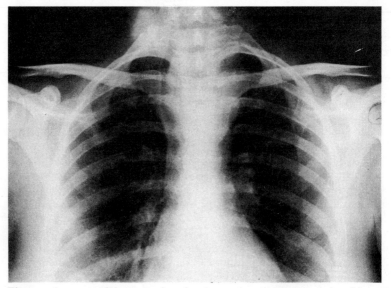

Fig. 7.1. An x-ray of thorax and neck, where a large retrosternal thyroid tumour is compressing and deviating the trachea to the right.

Position of patient

The position of the patient on the operating table is important. The head should be extended with the neck neither flexed or extended but in a neutral position.

Overextension of the neck can draw part of the thoracic trachea into the neck, and increase the likelihood of a low tracheostomy. This becomes embarrassingly evident at the end of the operation when the neck is flexed again.

Rotation of the head should be avoided because of anatomical distortion especially when other complications such as a local growth or obesity may make the distortion worse. A roll or sandbag is placed under the shoulders and a rubber ring or two sandbags should 'fix' the head (Fig. 7.2). The table should be tipped slightly head up, not only to increase accessibility for the surgeon but also to decrease venous distension.

Incision

The incision is a transverse collar incision approximately 50 mm long which is made 20 mm below the cricoid cartilage (Fig. 7.3). The classic vertical

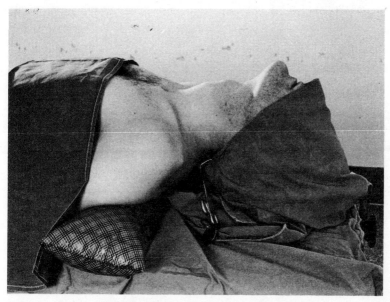

Fig. 7.2. Position for tracheostomy. Note the sandbag under the shoulders; the extended head should be supported on a rubber ring.

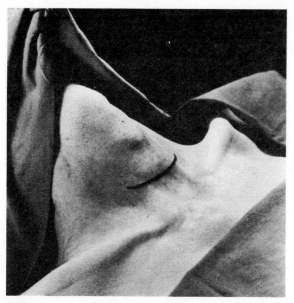

Fig. 7.3. Incision site for tracheostomy.

slit gives the advantage of draining well from the tract but scarring after closure is common. This can produce disfigurement and a heloid scar may limit chin movement.

Layers encountered

The reflected upper and lower edges are held apart with retractors while a vertical incision is made in the deep cervical fascia in the mid-line (Fig. 7.4). Beneath the fascia two muscles lie on each side, the sternohyoid

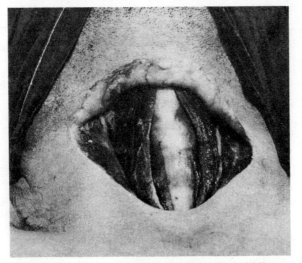

Fig. 7.4. The layers encountered. From the mid-line outwards one can see the medial edge of sternothyroid lying beneath the sternohyoid, and the large muscle mass on each side is the sternomastoid.

overlying the slimmer sternothyroid muscle. The two bellies of the sterno-hyoid muscles meet in the mid-line and should be parted to show the isthmus of the thyroid lying in front of the second, third and fourth cartilaginous rings of the trachea.

The pretracheal fascia encloses both lateral lobes and isthmus of the thyroid gland and stretches across the trachea in front above and below the isthmus. If the venous plexus within the fascia is engorged as in cases of obstruction to the airway, the isthmus of the thyroid is better divided. Normally, however, the isthmus can be retracted towards the head and the third and fourth rings of the trachea identified by palpation with the fore-finger (Fig. 7.5).

The level of the stoma to be made in the trachea is important. No incision should ever include the first cartilaginous ring. A perichondritis of the cricoid cartilage may result and certainly the risk of subglottic stenosis is considerable.

Incision of the trachea below the fourth ring is dangerous because the trachea lies deep and in close proximity to the great vessels of the neck,

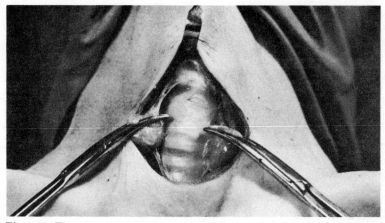

Fig. 7.5. The thyroid isthmus divided, showing the cricothyroid and first three tracheal rings.

including the left innominate vein. In addition, should the tracheostomy tube become displaced postoperatively, its replacement can be difficult and dangerous. Furthermore, the distance from the stoma to the bifurcation of the trachea is reduced, this is important when using a cuffed tracheostomy tube. Lastly, surgical emphysema is more common with a lower stoma. The stoma should thus be made at the level of the third and fourth rings, utilizing the second if the patient is short (Fig. 7.6).

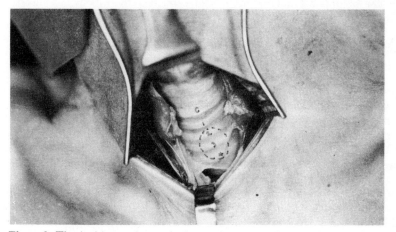

Fig. 7.6. The incision to be made for tracheostomy. C, cricoid cartilage; 1, 2, 3, tracheal rings.

The type of stoma

1. The so-called 'standard' tracheal stoma is a hole cut to the same size as the tracheal tube in the anterior wall of the trachea. An 11 or 15 surgical

blade may be used to incise the tracheal wall and cartilages, although when using a cuffed tube, extra pieces of third or fourth cartilaginous rings may have to be removed using a Citelli punch forceps (Fig. 7.7a).

2. The Bjork (1960) flap consists of an anterior tracheal flap raised from the second, third and fourth rings as illustrated (Fig. 7.7b). This flap is then sutured to the lower skin edge.

3. Hewlett and Ranger's method (1960) is to suture the lower skin edge to the lower margin of a 'standard' tracheal stoma.

4. The T-shaped incision (Nils–Gunnar Toremarn, 1974) is a vertical one through the third and fourth rings but joining above with a transcartilaginous slit in the second cartilage. The two edges are then held apart while the tube is inserted (Fig. 7.7c).

Haemostasis must be established at every stage, and it is common for the stomal edges to bleed from the cut cartilages on either side. Clinically, the postoperative course after tracheostomy is far less troublesome if the wound edges are dry.

The problems of types of tracheostomy

The different methods of performing a tracheostomy impose different problems during the management of tracheostomy.

The standard tracheal window is quick to perform. It causes little interference with laryngeal reflexes or coughing, and the tract closes quickly after extubation. The disadvantages are that replacement of the tube can be difficult and traumatic replacement of the tube is more likely.

Conversely, the methods of Bjork (1960) and Hewlett and Ranger (1960) provide a more easily identifiable tract and replacement is easy while displacement is less likely to occur. However, suturing and fixation of the trachea to the skin edges appears to make swallowing more difficult and an anterior flap may cause obstruction. Closure of the tract may be delayed and a planned operative closure may be required.

The T-shaped incision is designed to obviate the danger of stenosis. The second cartilage retains its shape and, although incised, none of the third or fourth cartilage is removed, thus keeping the original cartilaginous framework of the trachea intact. The blood supply to the cartilage is poor and so subsequent scarring is reduced to a minimum. Replacement of the tube is nevertheless difficult and dislodgement can occur.

Types of tracheostomy tubes

The types of tracheostomy tubes used (Fig. 7.8) will depend upon the indications for the operation and the prognosis arising from the underlying pathology. In the context of non-malignant conditions where the use of a prosthetic airway has a finite time limit, plastic cuffed tubes are used most frequently. Red rubber tubes can invite a considerable tissue reaction and the material itself is too rigid for long-term use. Plastic tubes tend to shape themselves to that of the airway at body temperature and the larger

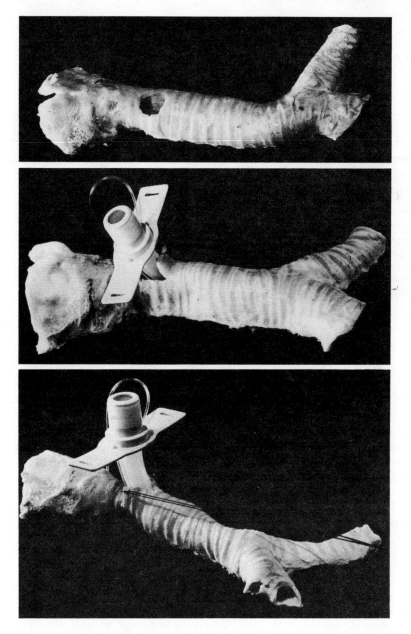

Fig. 7.7. Types of tracheostomy:

(a) standard incision;
(b) the Bjork flap with a tube in place;
(c) the T-shaped incision with a tube in place.

'floppy' cuff now commonly used can effect a sealed airway at a much reduced intracuff pressure (Crawley and Cross, 1975). Silver metal tubes are generally only used in postlaryngectomy situations, during the weaning period after prolonged ventilation or after acute exacerbations of obstructive airways disease. In these cases the most commonly used metal tube is the King's College Hospital (KCH) tracheal tube. This is especially useful because of the inclusion of a speaking tube. An appropriate one for a man is size 32 or 34 and size 28 for a woman.

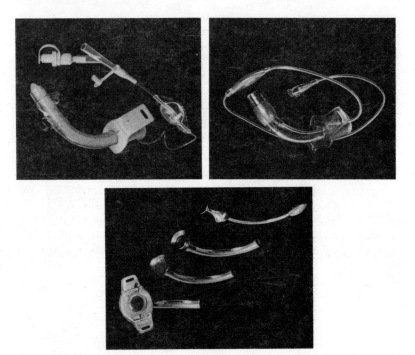

Fig. 7.8. A large-volume low-pressure, cuffed tracheostomy tube at the top left; a conventional tracheostomy tube at the top right; and a King's College Hospital (KCH) metal tracheostomy tube at the bottom with both introducer and speaking tube attachments.

The choice of tracheostomy tube

Where isolation of the airway from the pharynx is necessary

To reduce the incidence of tracheal mucosal damage following prolonged tracheal intubation it is now thought that the pressure exerted on the mucosa by the tracheal cuff should be as low as possible.

The perfusion pressure of the mucosal vessels is variously estimated at between 32 and 70 mm Hg (4·3 and 9·3 kPa). Ideally the tracheal wall pressure should be below this. This is now achieved by using large-volume low-pressure cuffs (Crawley and Cross, 1975). Here the cuff is not fully

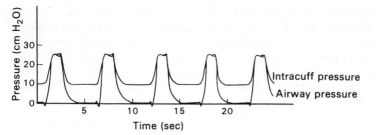

Fig. 7.9. Changes in airway and cuff pressure for a large-volume low-pressure, 'floppy' cuffed tracheostomy tube. The lower trace shows the machine or airway pressure, and the upper trace shows the changes in intracuff pressure associated with the respiratory cycle. Note that the cuff pressure never exceeds airway pressure. (From Crawley and Cross, 1975, *Anaesthesia*, **30**, 4.)

distended when effecting an airway seal and the intracuff pressure is equal to the tracheal wall pressure. When measured, the intracuff pressure generally follows airway pressure from the ventilator, and so a mean pressure of about 10–12 mm Hg (1·3–1·6 kPa) is achieved (Fig. 7.9).

$$P_{IC} = P_{TW} + P_{F(D+S)}$$

Intracuff pressure = Tracheal wall pressure + a pressure function of the 'floppy' cuff diameter and the compliance of the cuff material

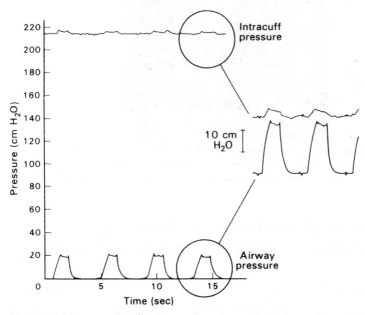

Fig. 7.10. Airway and cuff pressures in a conventional low-volume high-pressure, cuffed tracheostomy tube. Note that the intracuff pressure is very high and relatively unaffected by changes in airway pressure. (From Crawley and Cross, 1975, *Anaesthesia*, **30**, 4.)

Low-volume high-pressure cuffs (the so-called conventional cuff) tend to be fully distended and the tracheal wall pressure is the intracuff pressure less a function of the cuff diameter and the stiffness of the cuff material. In other words, some of the pressure within the cuff is counteracted by the elasticity of the cuff material, depending on how much it is distended. Thus, although the intracuff pressure in conventional cuffs commonly is measured as being as high as 180 mm Hg (24 kPa), the pressure applied to the tracheal wall varies. It has now been adequately demonstrated that low pressure or 'floppy' cuffs when correctly inflated can considerably reduce the incidence of tracheal injury (Cooper and Grillo, 1972) (Fig. 7.10).

Where the trachea has been separated from the pharynx surgically

Here (i.e. in the treatment of laryngeal tumours) intubation of the trachea is not necessary in order to control the airway to perform IPPV or to remove secretions. A tube is kept in place in these patients to prevent scarring reducing the operculum or stoma. The most useful example of this sort of tube is the KCH pattern, which is an admirable combination of the best features of many other designs (Fig. 7.11).

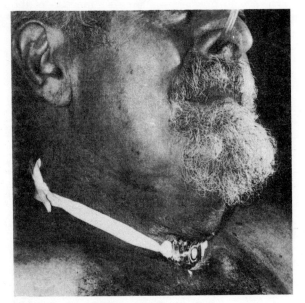

Fig. 7.11. The KCH metal tube in place.

References

Bjork, V. O. (1960). Partial resection of the only remaining lung with the aid of respirator treatment. *J. Thoracic Cardiovasc. Surg.*, **39**, 179.

Cooper, J. D. and Grillo, H. C. (1972). Analysis of problems relating to cuffs on intratracheal tubes. *Chest*, **62**, 21s.

Crawley, B. E. and Cross, D. E. (1975). Tracheal cuffs: a review and dynamic pressure study. *Anaesthesia*, **30**, 4.

Davison, M. H. Armstrong (1965). *The Evolution of Anaesthesia*. Sherratt, Altrincham.

Hewlett, A. B. and Ranger, D. (1960). Tracheostomy. *Postgrad. med. J.*, **37**, 18.

Lee, J. A. and Atkinson, R. S. (1973). *Synopsis of Anaesthesia*, 7th edn. John Wright, Bristol. pp. 142–3.

Toremarn Nils–Gunnar (1974). NLV Course, Malmö–lund.

Chapter 8

Complications of Tracheostomy

The insertion of an artificial prosthesis into the trachea cannot be performed without risk. Historically (Keys, 1945; Davison, 1965), an emergency tracheostomy was the very dramatic answer to terminal severe respiratory failure and the incidence of complications was overshadowed by the danger of the underlying disease. Today the patient is very frequently already intubated and the procedure of tracheostomy becomes an elective procedure performed at the surgeon's convenience and without stress. Under these conditions the complications of the procedure seem more relevant. Some of the complications can now be ameliorated or avoided by careful technique and stringent after-care. Although the incidence of complications is much reduced, when they do occur they are often associated with the underlying disease process which demanded the procedure of tracheostomy (Watts, 1963).

Operative complications

Haemorrhage

Venous bleeding at the time of the operation may be severe because respiratory obstruction, coughing or straining will all distend the neck veins.

Adequate haemostasis will not only prevent bleeding during and after the operation, but also reduce the incidence and severity of stomal infection.

Air embolus

Although rarely reported, air embolus may occur with any operation in the neck, due to damage to a large vein in the root of the neck.

Damage to nearby structures

This was more of a problem when emergency tracheostomy was the rule. Today, with the trachea supported in the mid-line by an indwelling endotracheal tube, the likelihood of damage to other nearby structures is reduced. It is, however, possible to damage or sever the vessels in the carotid sheath, the recurrent laryngeal nerve or even the oesophagus, and in children it has been reported that the pleura has been damaged.

Apnoea

Following the introduction of a prosthesis in the upper airway the dead space is much reduced and this may be responsible for the onset of apnoea a few minutes after the operation is completed. Since ventilatory monitoring is now the rule, it is unlikely that apnoea will be allowed to progress and produce cerebral damage or cardiac arrest.

Postoperative complications

Postoperative complications are both short and long term in nature. The short-term complications are as follows.

Wound infection

This is frequently found in conjunction with generalized infection, and *Streptococcus viridans* (α–*haemolytic streptococci*) or *Pseudomonas pyocyaneus* (*Pseudomonas aeruginosa*) are common infecting agents. Frequent toilet, clean dressings and control of respiratory secretions will often solve the problem.

Tracheitis

Trauma from suction catheters may cause inflammation and even ulceration of the tracheal mucosa. A separate sterile catheter should be used for every attempt at suction. This, together with humidification, should minimize this complication.

Blockage of the tracheostomy tube

This may occur if the tracheobronchial secretions are allowed to dry due to lack of humidification. Humidified inspired air at body temperature helps to preserve the ciliary activity of the tracheobronchial mucosa and to keep the secretions fluid. The instillation of 1–2 ml of sterile normal saline or sodium bicarbonate (2%) into the trachea before suction may be helpful. Great vigilance is necessary to guard against a tube becoming blocked, and any increase in respiratory effort by the patient, or undue restlessness, should always raise the possibility of this occurrence. Figure 8.1 shows a tracheostomy tube that has become blocked by secretions; the inner tube should be removed, inspected, cleaned and reinserted. If a rubber or plastic tube is in use, it should be cleaned by aspiration or changed for a new tube.

Obstruction to the airway may also be caused by overinflation and herniation of the cuff. This may occur transmurally into the lumen (DHSS, 1975) or the cuff may bulge over the tip of the tube. Intubation of the right main bronchus should also be borne in mind when investigating obstruction of the airway, especially when using double cuffed tubes in a short patient.

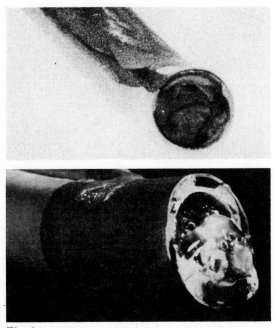

Fig. 8.1.

(a) A used KCH tracheostomy tube. Note the encrustation of the inner lumen.

(b) Cuffed tube sectioned to show blockage with mucus due to inadequate toilet.

Displacement of the tube

If the tapes securing the tracheostomy tube are too slack the tube may easily be coughed forward out of the tracheostome and the end may accidentally come to lie in the pretracheal tissues or outside the neck. In the former case the tube may not appear to be out of place and some air may pass down the track around the tube but respiratory obstruction rapidly increases. Double tapes of unequal length are a precaution against this serious accident. One pair is tied immediately the tube is inserted, while the patient's neck is still extended. When the neck is flexed its diameter is reduced and the second pair is then tied. The knots are at the side of the neck and cannot be mistaken for the knots of the patient's gown, and with two sets one knot may be adjusted at a time, so that the tube is never free for an instant. Should a suction catheter fail to pass freely into the trachea well beyond the end of the tracheostomy tube, it is possible that the tube is either blocked with secretions or is dislodged from the trachea. It should be removed and a new tube reinserted at once.

Subcutaneous emphysema of the neck

This condition may follow overtight suturing of the tracheostomy neck wound, emergency operations where there is acute respiratory distress (e.g.

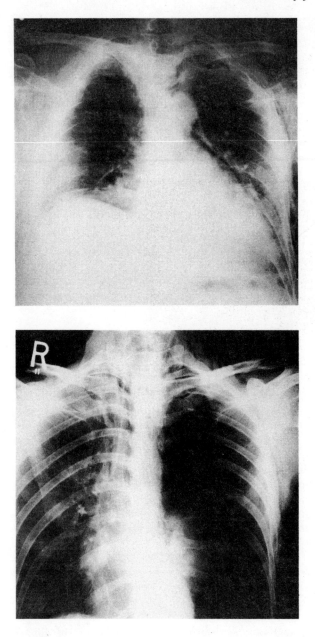

Fig. 8.2.

(a) The upper x-ray shows both mediastinal emphysema and subcutaneous emphysema. Note the air space surrounding the cardiac shadow.
(b) The lower x-ray shows a left pneumothorax pushing the mediastinal contents and the trachea to the right.

laryngotracheobronchitis), failure to intubate or bronchoscope infants preoperatively, and blockage or displacement of the tracheostomy tube. It is more common in children. On inspiration, air is drawn into the sub-cutaneous tissues and may be recognized as a swelling with a bubbling or crackling sensation palpable on light pressure.

However, subcutaneous emphysema very often does not arise from an overt trespass of the tracheal wall. Subcutaneous or mediastinal emphysema may result from previous trauma to the underlying lung tissues or from widespread lung infection. This may ultimately manifest itself as a tension pneumothorax. This triad of subcutaneous emphysema with spread into the mediastinum resulting in a pneumothorax in the absence of trauma to the lung can follow a prolonged period of IPPV if the inflation pressure needs to be high as in patients with interstitial oedema of the lung (Fig. 8.2). Drainage of the pleural cavity and aspiration of the air in the pleural cavity will often relieve the spreading emphysema for some time. Ultimately, however, the underlying disease process which required high-pressure IPPV has to be effectively treated.

In general the long-term complications fall under three main headings:

1. Laryngeal inco-ordination.
2. Damage to the tracheal wall.
3. Long-term scarring effects.

1. Laryngeal inco-ordination

This may be due in part to a long period of disuse and may lead to mild symptoms of hoarseness or dysphagia for a limited period of time. Dysphagia is not uncommon for the first few days after tracheostomy, due to inco-ordination of the swallowing mechanism. Infants often need tube-feeding. Cuffed tracheostomy tubes may press on the oesophagus through the soft posterior tracheal wall and cause an obstruction to swallowed food.

However, the re-education process may be slow and inco-ordination may also be associated with tethering of the trachea to the skin, and a loss of protective reflexes may result. This in turn may allow soiling of the tracheo-bronchial tree, giving rise to obstructive airways disease and sometimes an infective or chemical pneumonitis. An ineffective cough may produce an accumulation of secretions and if the patient becomes infected, a broncho-pneumonia or lobar pneumonia can occur.

2. Damage to the tracheal wall

Damage to the tracheal wall may be manifest in a number of different ways.

A mild tracheitis with oedema and inflammation. This may seem unimportant. However, in the presence of previous obstructive airways disease, secretion accumulation can lead to pulmonary infection.

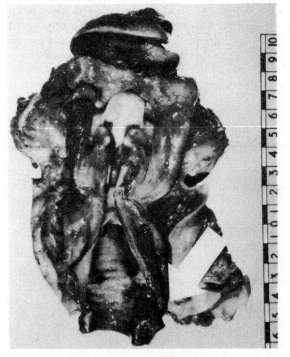

Fig. 8.3. Specimen of larynx and trachea, showing an erosion of the tracheal wall (arrowed) at the level of the balloon cuff. Erosion of the innominate artery caused fatal haemorrhage.

Ulceration. More severe damage to the tracheal wall resulting in ulceration can produce erosion of the tracheal wall. In an extreme case a fatal haemorrhage from ulceration into the innominate vein has been reported (Fig. 8.3).

Tracheomalacia. This is the result of pressure being applied to the cartilaginous rings of the trachea, usually in the presence of infection. Tracheomalacia and the resulting dilatation of the tracheal wall again may result in perforation of the tracheal wall into other structures; i.e. the oesophagus or a softened and weakened tracheal wall may allow air to pass into the surrounding tissues of the neck.

Adhesions and granuloma formation. Following both oedema and ulceration of the tracheal wall, adhesions may form within the airway, producing membranes across part or the whole of the airway. Local granulomas may be treated either by diathermy or excision but membranes hanging across the airway must be broken down and dilated with bronchial bougies. Very often membrane formation becomes a chronic process, and long periods of treatment are necessary.

Stenosis and collapse. The longer-term result of tracheal wall damage may be subglottic stenosis or tracheal wall collapse. The resulting narrowing of the upper airway is often distressing and ultimately, with infection, oedema and obstruction, may be fatal (Fig. 8.4). Subclinical, post-tracheostomy stenosis is surprisingly common.

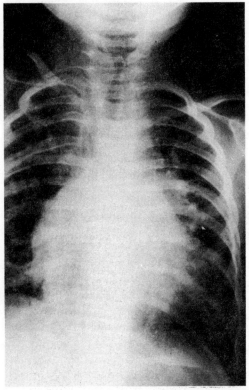

Fig. 8.4. This x-ray shows a subglottic stenosis of the trachea following prolonged intubation associated with a tracheo-oesophageal fistula.

Long-term scarring effects

Lastly, long-term scarring of the tracheostome can result in disfiguring scarring of the skin and underlying tissues. This may be associated with tethering of the trachea to other surrounding structures.

Aetiology of tracheal stenosis

Stenosis of the trachea may occur at three different sites: the stoma, the site of the cuff and opposite the distal tip of the tube. Numerous factors have been incriminated in the aetiology of the trauma to the trachea and its subsequent complications (Cooper and Grillo, 1960; Bassett, 1971). The composition, shape and size of endotracheal and tracheostomy tubes, movement of the tube and laryngeal activity often associated with IPPV have all been cited. Tracheo-oesophageal fistula and erosion of the innominate artery were among the earliest noted complications (Flege, 1967; Reich, 1968; Ivankovic et al., 1969). It was also associated with the technique of intermittent deflation of the cuff carried out over a prolonged period. With the discontinuation of this practice, a resultant fall in the incidence of ulceration and, ultimately, stenosis has resulted (English and Manley, 1970; Jenicek et al., 1973). The airway seal or cuff has been incriminated in tracheal trauma but it is only recently that the relationship between tracheal wall pressure and perfusion pressure within the tracheal mucous membrane has been emphasized. It is now recognized that low perfusion pressures in the tracheal wall as well as mucosal damage associated with factors such as thermal and chemical injuries and local infection will predispose to damage to the tracheal wall opposite the cuff. In addition, the danger of anticoagulant therapy have recently been emphasized. The more recent use of low-pressure or floppy cuffs has been shown to reduce considerably the incidence of tracheal injury when correctly inflated (Crawley and Cross, 1975) because the cuff pressure rarely rises above tracheal wall perfusion pressure (Fig. 8.5).

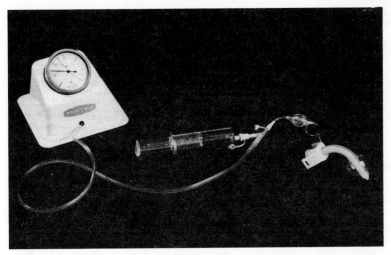

Fig. 8.5. A Portex 'soft seal' tracheostomy tube with a large-volume cuff and, on the left, a manometer showing a cuff pressure of 15 cm H_2O (1·5 kPa).

The ways of avoiding the complications of tracheostomy are as follows:

1. A meticulous surgical approach during the performance of tracheostomy with a controlled patient and a secure airway at all times.

2. The use of sterile techniques when handling the patient and, in particular, the tracheostome and the airway.

3. The use of sterile suction catheters and hand gloves whenever suction is performed.

4. Adequate parenteral nutrition and fluid balance. This is probably

more important than saturating the patient with excessive and overzealous humidification.

5. The sensible use of a large-volume low-pressure floppy cuff and the consequent use of lower tracheal wall pressures to effect an airway seal.

6. Stabilization of the tracheostomy tube, allowing less movement on moving the patient and during IPPV.

7. The prompt treatment of airway infection and hypotensive states.

8. The discontinuation of cuff deflation every 4 hours. This should only be necessary when changing the tube.

Realistically, the benefits of tracheostomy far outweigh the dangers and inconvenience of complications of the technique. It is well to remember that some respiratory infections can cause tracheal wall damage and produce surgical emphysema and a pneumothorax without intubation or tracheostomy being performed. Conversely, while tracheostomy can afford dramatic relief in some severe respiratory illnesses, it will not reverse an underlying disease process.

References

Bassett, H. F. M. (1971). Etiology of tracheal stenosis following cuffed intubation. *Proc. roy. Soc. Med.*, **64**, 890.

Cooper, J. D. and Grillo, H. C. (1969). The evolution of tracheal injury due to ventilatory assistance through cuffed tubes: a pathologic study. *Ann. Surg.*, **169**, 334.

Crawley, B. E. and Cross, D. E. (1975). Tracheal cuffs: a review and dynamic pressure study. *Anaesthesia*, **30**, 4.

DHSS (1975). *A Problem with Plastic Cuffed Endotracheal Tubes.* CMO 9/75 (24-3-75).

Davison, M. H. Armstrong (1965). *The Evolution of Anaesthesia.* Sherratt, Altrincham.

English, I. C. W. and Manley, R. E. W. (1970). The Brompton system of artificial ventilation. A scheme for the intensive care unit. *Anaesthesia*, **25**, 541.

Flege, J. B. Jr. (1967). Tracheoesophageal fistula caused by cuffed tracheostomy tube. *Ann. Surg.*, **166**, 153.

Ivankovic, A. D. *et al.* (1969). Fatal haemorrhage from the innominate artery after tracheostomy. A case report. *Brit. J. Anaesth.*, **41**, 450.

Jenicek, J. A. *et al.* (1973). Continuous cuff inflation during long term intubation and ventilation: evaluation and technique. *Anaesth. Analg. Curr. Res.*, **52**, 252.

Keys, Thomas E. (1945). *The History of Surgical Anesthesia.* Schuman, New York.

Reich, M. P. (1968). Fistula between innominate artery and trachea. *Archs Surg. (Chicago)*, **96**, 401.

Watts, J. McK. (1963). Tracheostomy in modern practice. *Brit. J. Surg.*, **50**, 954.

Chapter 9

Management of a Tracheostomy

Introduction

The benefits of a tracheostomy in the treatment of respiratory failure may well be lost if the postoperative care is inadequate. Most of the serious complications of tracheostomy occur within the first few days of operation (Watts, 1963), and the risks can be minimized by careful and skilled attention during this period.

Pre-operative measures

If the patient is conscious and understands the significance of his pathology then every attempt should be made to explain why the operation is being performed and what effect this will have on his normal functions. It is also wise at this point to plan how to amuse and entertain the patient postoperatively together with providing the means of communication (warning bells, lights, pencil and paper, etc.) It is as important to supply visual and audible interests (i.e. radio, television and books) as it is to give an adequate and varied diet.

Care during the immediate postoperative period

The hazards which may occur immediately postoperatively are as follows:

1. The airway may be obstructed by blood from the wound edges or by pharyngeal contents and secretions from the lower respiratory tract.

2. The tube may become displaced.

3. The respiratory pattern may change following the introduction of an artificial airway, with diminution of dead space and a decrease in airways resistance.

4. Surgical emphysema and pneumothorax.

During this post-tracheostomy period the patient must continue to be monitored and the original pathology must continue to be treated. A trained nurse must be in attendance for 24 hours per day until the patient is able to look after his own airway. If the patient is to be artificially ventilated the nurse must be conversant with the mechanism of the ventilator and know what action to take should the machine fail.

At the bedside

At the bedside there must be:

1. A powerful and efficient sucker with an adequate supply of sterile non-traumatic suction catheters; the diameter of these catheters should be less than half the diameter of the tracheostomy tube.

2. A supply of disposable gloves.

3. A pair of tracheostomy dilators.

4. A spare tracheostomy tube of similar size and pattern to that already in place.

5. A laryngoscope and endotracheal tube to be used in the event of unsuccessful replacement of the tracheostomy tube.

6. A good portable light.

7. A bell for summoning assistance.

8. A pencil and paper for the conscious patient.

9. A means of alternative manual ventilation; e.g. a self-inflating bag together with an expiratory valve, a catheter mount and a readily available oxygen supply.

10. A Wright respirometer or similar apparatus for measuring the minute and tidal volumes.

The general management of a tracheostomy

The general management of a tracheostomy must include the following:

1. The monitoring, assessment and provision of adequate ventilation (Fig. 9.1).

2. The monitoring of vital functions, e.g. ECG, blood pressure and fluid balance (Fig. 9.1).

3. The instigation of drug regimens for sedation, analgesia, control of infection, etc.

4. Nutrition given orally, via a nasogastric tube or by intravenous infusion.

5. Care of bladder function, with catheterization if necessary.

6. General care for eyes, ears, mouth, rectum, etc.

7. Frequent change of position, and skin care.

8. Physiotherapy for musculoskeletal function and drainage of airway secretions, pus, etc.

Problems related to tracheostomy and their management

The upper airway has a number of important functions which are lost when an artificial prosthesis is inserted into the trachea (Slome, 1971).

The nose, nasopharynx and pharynx have the following functions:

1. Warming the inspired air from ambient temperature up to approximately 34° C in the trachea. The lining membrane of the upper respiratory tract has an abundant blood supply spread over a considerable surface area, and the folds of this membrane act as a very efficient heating element.

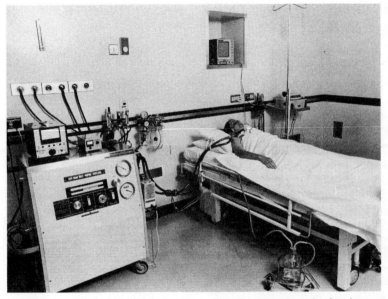

Fig. 9.1. A general view of a patient in an intensive therapy unit, showing monitoring arrangements and ventilation attachments.

2. Humidifying the inspired air.

3. Filtering the inspired air and trapping particulate matter in the mucous and serous secretions produced by the upper respiratory tract.

Without the nose and pharynx, the inspired air would be cold, dry and unfiltered. Obstruction of the airway would be more likely because secretions would become drier and more difficult to remove. Also, a shorter direct route would be provided for infection.

Methods of humidification

The three main methods of humidification are:

1. Conservation of exhaled water vapour
2. Heated water reservoirs
3. Nebulization

1. Conservation of heat and water content of the exhaled air

These can be retained to some extent using a condenser/humidifier (Fig. 9.2). The condenser may be in the form of a wire mesh or as a folded paper gauze. During expiration exhaled water condenses on to the filter and the heat of the expired gas is retained within the condenser. As the inspired gas passes over the mesh it is warmed up and picks up the retained water content. The metal gauze humidifiers are quite effective but also heavy. The corrugated paper plugs in a plastic shell are lighter and, for this reason, to be preferred. They are more effective (Bethune and Walker, 1976) and in addition, because of their cheapness, they can be replaced. While the filter will also trap organisms, this will not prove a danger if they are replaced at frequent intervals.

The main disadvantages are that in patients where a dry gas is added to the condenser (i.e. oxygen) their humidifying function is far less efficient

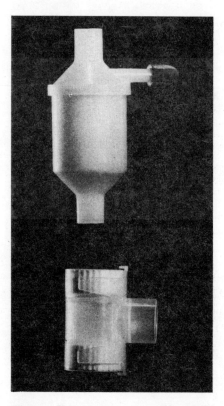

Fig. 9.2. Two condenser/humidifiers. At the top is a Swedish attachment with a side arm to allow added oxygen to be given. At the bottom is a disposable, lightweight, condenser/humidifier with the cross-arm packed with corrugated paper.

and secretions can become viscid. This also occurs if the patient is dyspnoeic. Here the rate of inspiratory and expiratory flow increases through the humidifier with less opportunity for conservation of heat and water. The resistance of the condenser, which under experimental conditions is very low, can be greatly increased by the accumulation of secretions in the mesh. This underlines the importance of replacing this sort of humidifier every 3–4 hours. Its use in very young children is not advised because although the dead space increase is not important in adults, it can be very significant in young children. The increase in airways resistance with accumulated secretions could also assume importance in the very young.

2. Heated water reservoirs

The second method of humidifying inspired gases is by entraining the gas over a heated water reservoir. This is commonly used and relatively efficient. If the patient is being ventilated the machine pushes air, with or without additional dry gases such as oxygen, over a water reservoir which is heated by a thermostatically controlled electric element. The tubing connecting the humidifier to the patient should be as short as possible and have a very low heat conductivity. In addition, there should be a water trap into which condensed water can drain. Either the water temperature of the reservoir is kept at a higher temperature than 34° C in order to offset the inevitable heat loss down the inspiratory tubing to the patient or the inspiratory tubing may be heated.

If the patient is breathing spontaneously then the gas mixture to be inspired is blown over the heated water reservoir by a low resistance fan (Fig. 9.3). This provides an output of some 20–25 litres per minute which is blown across the top of the artificial airway in a T-piece or perforated plastic box. The temperature of the reservoir is kept higher than 34° C—at about 45–48° C—and the length and type of tubing is selected for the maximum conservation of the heat.

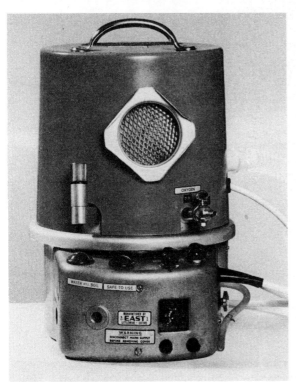

Fig. 9.3. An East blower/humidifier. Note the arrangements on the base to allow the contents to be boiled, thus making the unit self-disinfecting.

In addition to the electricity and temperature warning lights, the humi-difier can be separated from the patient and the contents boiled by adjust-ing the heating control. This enables it to be disinfected easily and fre-quently without disrupting the routine. The temperature of the inspired gas should be monitored as near to the patient as possible, it should not exceed 34° C. Higher temperatures can produce an unexplained pyrexia, especially in children.

3. Nebulization

The third method of humidification is to add microdroplets of water to the inspired gas by one of a number of methods. The life and effectiveness of the droplets depends on their size in the mist and the relative humidity of the carrier gas (Robinson, 1974). The larger water particles have a smaller surface to volume ratio and thus less is lost in evaporation, which is also reduced by a high relative humidity. A high relative humidity will prolong the life of a droplet and this fact is used in some humidifiers to increase their efficiency. The benefit derived from humidification depends upon the size of the droplets. Initially, when generated, large droplets of 10–20 μm tend to be baffled by the walls of the container. The depth of penetration down the respiratory tree will also depend on the size of the droplet. Ideally, it is necessary to produce a broad scan of droplets from 2 to 15 μm in size and to have a total water content in the inspired air of 44 mg/l. This is the water content of saturated air at a temperature of 37° C. Microdroplets are produced by nebulizers which may be either ultrasonic or gas driven.

Ultrasonic nebulizers produce an aerosol of water droplets by oscillating a diaphragm at a very high frequency beneath a layer of water (Fig. 9.4). The droplet size tends to be uniform and at the lower end of the scale (i.e. 2–10 μm). They produce a high water content and can easily produce a supersaturated gas. This has disadvantages as it increases the airways resistance and may give rise to water intoxication, especially in infants. Gas-driven nebulizers produce their water particles by using a high pressure jet of gas to suck up a fine column of water into the gas stream and to project it on to a curved surface, thereby causing the water to break up into very fine particles. The range of droplets produced is wide, from 2 to 30 μm, and a large number of the bigger particles are baffled in the container and tubing. This gas leaves the nebulizer with a low mist density and a relatively low water content (e.g. 20–35 mg/l). However, some gas-driven nebulizers have a heated water reservoir and, because this raises the relative humidity of the carrier gas, it increases the life of the nebulized droplets, and so increases the water content. A good example of this type of nebulizer is the Ohio (Fig. 9.5).

Other methods

(a) The steam kettle is an electrically heated water reservoir which produces steam at the end of a fan-shaped spout. It raises the relative humidity of the environment a little.

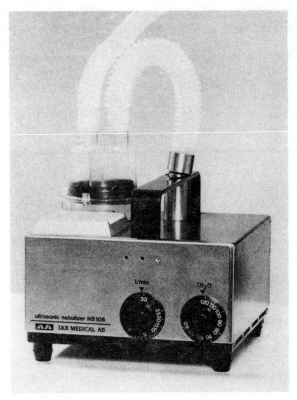

Fig. 9.4. LKB ultrasonic nebulizer. The two controls allow a change in flow rate and water content.

(b) Bubbling the inspired gas through a water reservoir (i.e. the Wolfe bottle) is ineffectual in raising the water content of the gas.

(c) A saline drip given intermittently into a tracheostomy tube is inaccurate and may have tragic results if constant attention is not provided.

There has been considerable discussion recently about the supposed need for humidification. Some authorities would argue that metaplastic change in the trachea—that is, the changing of the lining cells from a ciliated columnar epithelium to a squamous epithelium—takes place within 3–4 days. At the end of this time the trachea and main bronchi are serving the function of the nose and pharynx while there is increased secretory function below this level. If this is so, why put the patient to a risk of infection which is not strictly necessary? It is argued that it is better to use intermittent injection of saline down the trachea during the first 3–4 days and after this humidification will not be necessary.

The reservoirs of the humidifiers constitute a major source of infection in the intensive therapy unit and are therefore a potential hazard to the patient. Some would argue that, in patients with increased secretory activity, the use of dry gas will encourage the formation of secretions and

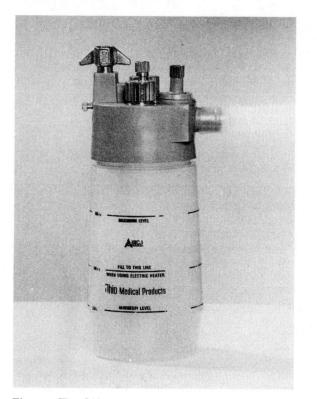

Fig. 9.5. The Ohio gas nebulizer. A heating element may be inserted to raise the relative humidity of the carrier gas.

respiratory obstruction. The middle of the road approach may well be a sensible answer; i.e. those who need humidification should be provided with adequately sterilized reservoirs of humidified water but in general more patients should be encouraged to do without.

Routine care of the tracheostomy wound

If the wound becomes infected a bacterial swab should be taken, the organisms and sensitivities determined and the appropriate antibiotic administered. A dry dressing may be placed on the wound and changed every 24 hours, or more frequently if it becomes very soiled.

Securing the tracheostomy tube

Displacement of the tube is one of the many ways in which loss of a patent airway occurs and may easily be prevented by correct fixation. Two sets of tapes 13 mm wide attached to the tracheostomy tube should be looped round the patient's neck and tied with a reef knot and bow on each side of the neck. If the tapes are too loose the tube is liable to become displaced. If they are too tight or the knot is placed posteriorly the patient suffers discomfort. The correct tension of the tapes is obtained by securing the knot when the head is held in a slightly flexed position. If possible, the tube should remain undisturbed initially for 5–7 days so that an adequate tract forms. Coloured tape should be used to secure the tracheostomy to distinguish them from the tapes of the patient's gown.

Care of the airway

The larynx has three main functions:

1. Protection of the airway from pharyngeal contents, foreign bodies, etc.

2. To allow an explosive evacuation of the airway by suddenly releasing a closed glottis.

3. Phonation and communication.

The last function has already been dealt with earlier in this chapter. The protection and clearing of the airway is the most important function of respiratory care.

Removal of secretions

The presence of secretions is inevitable in the initial stages of a tracheostomy, particularly if the operation is performed on a patient with chronic lung disease. In addition, the tube acts as a foreign body and stimulates secretions, whilst in the immediate postoperative period there may be some ooze of blood from the operation site. Removal of these secretions may be assisted by (1) coughing, (2) aspiration, and (3) cleaning or changing the tube.

1. Coughing

An explosive cough is not possible in the patient with a tracheostomy as pressure cannot be built up against a closed glottis. However, most conscious patients are able to bring their secretions up as far as the tracheostomy tube where aspiration is easily accomplished. The assistance of a physiotherapist is invaluable in training these patients to cough correctly (Fig. 9.6).

2. Aspiration

This is the only efficient method of secretion removal in the unconscious patient and must be performed regularly and efficiently (Fig. 9.7). Aspiration should be performed:

(a) if secretions can be heard rattling in the trachea;
(b) if it is required by the patient;
(c) if it is indicated by clinical examination of the chest;
(d) before and after turning the patient and also before deflation of the tracheal cuff.

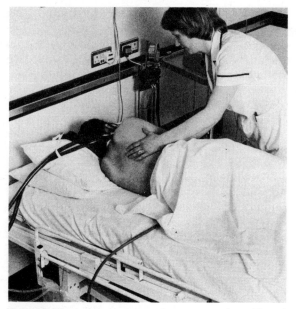

Fig. 9.6. Physiotherapy being given to a patient. Note that the bed head is tilted down to aid postural drainage.

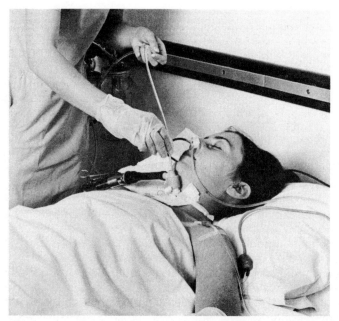

Fig. 9.7. Routine suction being carried out. Note the aseptic technique.

In the immediate postoperative period, aspiration may have to be carried out at shorter intervals (5–10 minutes) but this period may be lengthened as secretions become less in quantity, when 4-hourly aspiration may be adequate. Occasionally, if secretions become encrusted on the tracheal wall, they may have to be removed with forceps through a tracheoscope. Instillation of a few drops of 5% sodium bicarbonate solution into the trachea may assist in the removal of stubborn secretions. Aspiration should be carried out as follows.

The nurse wears a mask and, having washed her hands for 2 minutes with soap and water, puts a disposable glove on her right hand. A suitable, sterile, non-traumatic catheter is selected, the sucker is switched on with her left hand and the catheter, held by the gloved hand, is now advanced 150–230 mm into the tracheostomy tube, ensuring that it reaches as far as the carina. The thumb of the ungloved hand is now placed over the open limb of the Y-connection and the sputum aspirated, rotating the catheter as it is withdrawn. The manoeuvre should not take more than 10 seconds since, if this time is exceeded, it may render the patient hypoxic as the suction will prevent air reaching the alveoli. The catheter is now discarded into a bowl of sodium bicarbonate solution and a fresh catheter used for the next aspiration. It is most important that the diameter of the suction catheter should not be more than half the diameter of the tracheostomy tube because dangerous intrapulmonary negative pressure may be developed. This is particularly important in small children.

3. Cleaning the tracheostomy tube

Secretions may be deposited inside the tube and dry to form a crust despite all efforts to prevent it. Silver tracheostomy tubes possess a separate inner tube; secretions are thus easily removed by taking out the inner tube and substituting a fresh one. Initially, the inner tube must be changed every half-hour for cleaning and resterilizing, but this period may be prolonged to 4 hours as secretions diminish. With cuffed rubber and plastic tubes there is no removable inner tube and if secretions cause obstruction in these cases, the whole tube should be removed and a new one inserted.

Changing the tracheostomy tube

Cuffed tubes should be changed every 7 days or earlier if it is thought that the lumen has been decreased by encrusted secretions. The substitution should be carried out as a sterile procedure. The patient is placed in a supine, head-down position with the neck extended. The trachea and pharynx are aspirated before deflation of the cuff, the tapes securing the tube are cut and the tube removed. The tracheostome is quickly cleaned, a fresh tube inserted and the cuff inflated with sufficient air to provide an airtight fit. When introducing the new tube, the end inserted into the patient must be directed posteriorly through the stoma before it is turned caudally to pass down the lumen of the trachea. Failure to do so may result in placing the tube in the mediastinum anterior to the trachea. In the apnoeic patient, the change of tube should be accomplished rapidly so that minimal hypoxia occurs. Where difficulty in replacing a tracheostomy tube is anticipated, a laryngoscope, endotracheal tube and a means of inflating the patient should always be at hand. Following insertion of a new tracheostomy tube it is essential to auscultate the lungs to ensure both are expanding equally.

Care of the inflatable cuff

The cuff should be inflated with sufficient air to form an airtight seal with the tracheal wall, and the quantity of air required should be recorded on a chart. Should the cuff be deflated, it is important that it is fully deflated before the same amount of air is reintroduced. This is because most plastic cuffs do not shrink to their former shape; there is a residual volume of air left within the cuff. This residual volume tends to become larger with each subsequent inflation, deflation and so forth. The resulting overinflation of the cuff may result in:

    1. ischaemia and necrosis of the tracheal mucosa;
    2. pressure necrosis of the cartilaginous rings of the trachea;
    3. herniation of the cuff over the end of the tube, causing obstruction of the airway.

On the other hand, underinflation of the cuff allows pharyngeal secretions to leak into the lungs and may also render ventilation inadequate because of a gas leak. The cuff should not be deflated unless:

    1. the tube is to be replaced;
    2. the type of tube is changed; or
    3. the physician in charge requests it.

When this is done the patient should be in the head-down position and the pharynx and trachea aspirated before letting down the cuff. If the patient is being artificially ventilated the minute volume must be checked and the necessary adjustments made to the machine to maintain the correct minute volume. The cuff is then inflated until an effective airtight seal is reached. If the large-volume floppy cuff tube is being used, the intracuff pressure can be monitored on a manometer and this should always be below the ventilator airway pressure; i.e. 8–15 mm Hg (Cooper and Grillo, 1972).

Decannulation

When a patient is able to breathe spontaneously, without distress, maintaining his blood-gas levels within normal limits and is also able to swallow, his cuffed tube should be removed and a non-cuffed one substituted. Later, the lumen of this tube can be occluded by a cork so that all respirations now pass through the normal respiratory channels. If this added dead space is well tolerated, the tube should be removed and the stoma allowed to close. A large dry dressing applied to the tracheostome with waterproof strapping is all that is required whilst waiting for the stoma to close. Occasionally, it may be considered necessary to perform a surgical closure of the stoma for cosmetic reasons.

References

Bethune, D. W. and Walker, A. K. Y. (1976). A comparative study of condenser humidifiers. *Anaesthesia*, **31**, (no. 8), 1086.

Cooper, J. D. and Grillo, H. C. (1972). Analysis of problems related to cuffs on intratracheal tubes. *Chest*, **62**, 21s.

Robinson, J. S. (1974). In: *Scientific Foundations of Anaesthesia*, 2nd edn., p. 488. Ed. by C. F. Scurr and S. A. Feldman. Heinemann Medical, London.

Slome, D. (1971). In: *Scott Brown's Diseases of the Ear, Nose and Throat*, 3rd edn., Vol. 1, *Basic Sciences*, pp. 147, 235, 339. Ed. by J. C. Ballantyne and J. Groves. Butterworths, London and Boston, Mass.

Watts, J. McK. (1963). Tracheostomy in modern practice. *Brit. J. Surg.*, **1**, 954.

Chapter 10

Automatic Ventilators

Respiration consists of oxygen utilization and carbon dioxide and water production by cellular metabolism, and of necessity includes the transport of gases to and from the cell.

Ventilation is part of the transport mechanism which, together with the circulation, effects an exchange of oxygen and carbon dioxide. Ventilation is the intermittent inflation of the lungs with a respirable gas. This is normally performed by the muscles of respiration.

When ventilation is performed by an external force (i.e. mouth-to-mouth resuscitation, manual ventilation or by a machine), the end result should be the same as with spontaneous ventilation, and respirable gas should flow in and out of the lungs in a manner similar to normal ventilation.

Apart from the Drinker ventilator (iron lung) and cuirass, which create a negative pressure outside the chest wall and suck air into the patient, most ventilators in clinical use are positive pressure ventilators.

Positive pressure ventilators

Positive pressure ventilators are numerous and vary in their mode of function. Because of this, a number of classifications have been produced to clarify their mechanical working and performance in order to help the clinician (Hunter, 1961; Mapleson, 1962).

Classification

1. Ventilators may be classed according to their mode of delivery of gas to the patient's airway (Fig. 10.1). If the gas arrives at the airway at a constant flow regardless of the pressure developed and regardless of changes in airway resistance and lung compliance, then this type of ventilator is termed a **flow generator**. With this type of apparatus, if an obstruction to the airway develops, the machine will tend to overcome the obstruction irrespective of the pressure developed. In practice, all ventilators of this type have a safety valve which is preset at 50–70 cm H_2O (5–7 kPa).

If gas arrives at the patient's airway at a defined pressure regardless of the flow developed or changes in lung characteristics, then the machine is called a **pressure generator**; such a machine will tend to compensate for any leak in the airway or gas circuit but, faced with an increasing airways

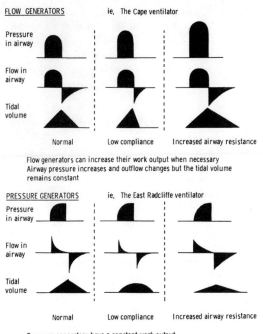

FLOW GENERATORS   ie, The Cape ventilator

Pressure
in airway

Flow in
airway

Tidal
volume

Normal   Low compliance   Increased airway resistance

Flow generators can increase their work output when necessary
Airway pressure increases and outflow changes but the tidal volume
remains constant

PRESSURE GENERATORS   ie, The East Radcliffe ventilator

Pressure
in airway

Flow in
airway

Tidal
volume

Normal   Low compliance   Increased airway resistance

Pressure generators have a constant work output
Airway pressure remains constant but tidal volume will fall and flow
will alter

Fig. 10.1. Characteristics of flow and pressure generators.

resistance or low compliance, the tidal volume delivered will decrease.

2. Another classification is to argue that since by definition all ventilators must cycle from inspiration to expiration they may be classified by their method of cycling; i.e. volume, time or pressure cycling (Fig. 10.2).

A time-cycled ventilator will cycle from inspiration to expiration when a predetermined·time has passed. In addition, this same ventilator may also be pressure preset; i.e. although the machine will only cycle when a

(1) Time-cycled ventilators Electronic————Barnet ventilator
                                Electromechanical—East Radcliffe ventilator
                                        —Cape ventilator
                                        —Engstrom   } volume
                                            ventilator } preset

(2) Pressure-cycled ventilators——Blease (can function as a volume preset machine)
                                     —Bird ventilator
                                     —Harlow ventilator

(3) Volume-cycled ventilators—Barnet Mark III ventilator

Fig. 10.2. Classification of ventilators by their method of ending inspiration. The Cape and the Engstrom ventilators have powerful electric motors that can produce a preset volume of gas regardless of any other parameter.

predetermined time has been reached, the pressure developed in the airway will not rise above a preset value. In this case it will be seen that with both time and pressure delineated, inspiratory flow and volume will vary and will be determined by the airway resistance and the lung compliance.

In the same way, a pressure- or volume-cycled ventilator will cycle from inspiration to expiration when a predetermined volume or pressure has been produced by the machine.

Although these methods of classification have their uses, in clinical practice it is better to have a working knowledge of the mechanical principles underlying the performance of the particular machine in use. It is more important to know how the machine functions, what its limits and disadvantages are and how it will behave when the external conditions alter.

To understand the mechanical working of a ventilator may be difficult with the sophisticated third and fourth generation models available. There are, however, only four important facets which must be known in order to achieve a reasonable working knowledge of the machine (Fig. 10.3).

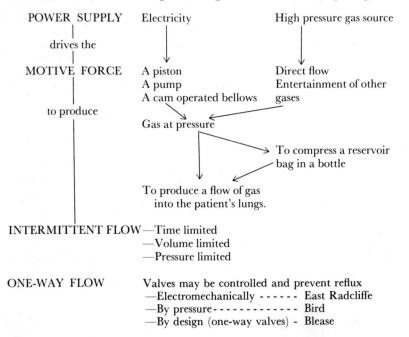

POWER SUPPLY — Electricity — High pressure gas source

drives the

MOTIVE FORCE — A piston / A pump / A cam operated bellows — Direct flow / Entertainment of other gases

to produce

Gas at pressure

To compress a reservoir bag in a bottle

To produce a flow of gas into the patient's lungs.

INTERMITTENT FLOW—Time limited
—Volume limited
—Pressure limited

ONE-WAY FLOW — Valves may be controlled and prevent reflux
—Electromechanically - - - - - - East Radcliffe
—By pressure - - - - - - - - - - - - Bird
—By design (one-way valves) - Blease

Fig. 10.3.

The power supply

The supply may be either electricity or a high-pressure gas source or both. For instance, the Barnet ventilator uses pressurized gas to fill the inflating bellows, and electricity to operate the electronically controlled solenoids which act as inspiratory and expiratory valves. The power supply may be used in a variety of ways to provide a motive force.

The motive force

This is used to provide gas at a higher pressure than in the lungs and to bring it to the upper airway. Electricity may drive an air pump, a piston in an enclosed cylinder, or a rotating cam to raise or compress an inflating bellows; alternatively, high gas pressure may be used to provide respirable gas through a reducing valve direct to the patient, to compress a reservoir bag or to raise an inflating bellows.

Cycling

All ventilators must produce an intermittent flow of gas. Flow of gas into the lungs must be interrupted and deflation allowed to occur.

Time cycling

This may be electromechanical. The most common method is by means of a rotating cam which, whilst not influenced by pressure or volume attained in the gas circuit, is related to the frequency of ventilation.

With such an arrangement there is almost always a fixed inspiratory–expiratory ratio; i.e. Cape, Engstrom and East Radcliffe ventilators. Time cycling may also be achieved by electronically controlled solenoids operating the expiratory valve as in the Loosco infant ventilator, or both inspiratory and expiratory valves as in the Barnet ventilator.

Pressure cycling

Here a preset pressure valve cycles the machine. Cycling occurs when this pressure is reached at a pressure-sensitive valve. This principle is used in the Blease Pulmoflator, the Bird and Harlow ventilators.

Volume cycling

This is unusual as a method of cycling and is usually confused with a volume preset mode of function. The Barnet Mark III can be used as a volume-cycled apparatus. 'Servo' ventilators deliver a preset flow rate and the inspiratory time can be varied. In effect this serves as a volume cycled machine. Examples are the Elema Siemens and BOC Pneumotron. In these examples the ventilatory waveform can be varied, though clinical use of this facility is doubtful.

One-way flow

This is achieved by one-way valves in both inspiratory and expiratory limbs. The most important point is that the expiratory valve must be held closed during inspiration. This may be achieved electronically as in the Barnet ventilator, electromechanically with rotating cams as in the East Radcliffe, or by connecting the valve to the pressure developed in the inspiratory line of the machine as in the Bird ventilator.

Knowledge of these four characteristics will enable the clinician using the machine to understand more fully the versatility and limits of the ventilators in practical use.

Choice of ventilator

The type of machine selected must depend largely upon the variety of functions it must serve and who is going to use it. The ideal ventilator would be small, disposable, sterile, versatile and very cheap. It has yet to be marketed. In practice, a ventilator which is to be used for patients with changing airways resistance and compliance as in chronic bronchitis and pulmonary oedema must be versatile and capable of producing a preset volume without regard to the pressure developed or changes in pulmonary characteristics. It should also need little supervision, and leave the staff free to devote their attention to the patient. These ventilators, which are usually time cycled and volume preset, are invariably large, expensive, difficult to clean and sterilize, and are mechanically sophisticated with too many controls. Nevertheless, they are the best machines in difficult clinical situations. Apart from this the choice of ventilator is a personal selection. But the following points may help to choose the best machine for the prevailing situation.

1. Simplicity. There should be as few controls as possible and they should be accessible and grouped together. Indicators should show accurate values of pressure in the airway and the volume delivered and not arbitrary figures with no meaning. These suggestions are important when the machine is to be used by staff of varying experience.

2. There should be an alternative form of ventilation through the machine in case of mechanical or power failure.

3. Versatility. It should be possible to provide air or oxygen enrichment or to use the machine to give anaesthetic gas mixtures.

4. Reliability. There should be warning devices in case of failure.

5. It should be as small as possible, without affecting its performance.

6. It should be possible to sterilize the patient's circuit including the expiratory valve, and in addition to make the rest of the machine domestically clean.

7. There should be a 24-hour servicing and replacement facility.

8. There should be easy access to the mechanical part of the ventilator in order to correct minor faults and for one's own instruction.

9. The machine should have provision for humidification of inspired gases.

10. It should be quiet in operation.

Artificial ventilation is not to be undertaken lightly, as it carries a morbidity and mortality rate. If the clinician is prepared to ventilate a patient he must understand the mechanical function of the machine to be used, and also appreciate the physiological changes produced by positive pressure ventilation.

There now follows a brief and simple description of seven commonly used ventilators.

The East Radcliffe ventilator (Fig. 10.4)

This ventilator is a constant-pressure generator. The pressure applied to the airway depends upon the adjustment of a weight on the inspiratory bellows. It is also a time-cycled machine, and so the tidal volume delivered to the patient will depend upon adjustment of the weight, the pulmonary characteristics of the patient, and the inspiratory time. A simple description of the mechanical working of the ventilator is as follows.

The power supply is electricity and this is used to drive an electric motor which rotates a geared cam shaft. The eccentric cam raises a pivoted arm upon which is an adjustable weight. The motive force is the compression of the inflatable bellows by the weight. Gas is drawn into the inflating bellows through a one-way valve by expansion of the bellows caused by the rotating cam. The cam shaft, in addition to providing the motive force, also opens and closes the inspiratory valve. Thus the machine is time cycled with a fixed inspiratory and expiratory ratio. Although this ratio is fixed the inspiratory time is altered when the frequency of ventilation is changed by altering the gear ratios between the electric motor and the cam shaft. One-way flow is achieved by valves operated by the cam shaft and it will be obvious that this type of machine cannot be triggered by the patient. There is also a spring-loaded expiratory bellows which can provide an optional negative phase during expiration.

The Cape Bristol ventilator (Fig. 10.5)

The Cape Bristol ventilator is a two-stage constant-volume flow generator. An electromechanical piston pump acts as a pressure generator and supplied air to the second-stage ventilating head. The head carries a self-inflating bellows within a transparent chamber which is compressed by the first-stage pump. Thus the bellows acts as a preset constant-volume flow generator. The volume delivered to the patient is adjusted by altering the excursion of the bellows. Inspiratory flow can be varied and there is a fixed inspiratory–expiratory timing ratio of $1:2$. The timing is controlled by a mechanical cam-operated poppet valve in time with the piston.

The Cape multi-purpose ventilator (Fig. 10.5)

This ventilator is a constant-flow generator. It is time cycled and volume preset. The power source is electricity driving a powerful motor. Gas enters the inspiratory bellows through a one-way valve and the bellows is compressed directly by a rocking arm driven by the motor. The tidal volume can be adjusted by altering the pivot of this rocking arm. The machine is time cycled in that both the inspiratory and expiratory valves are controlled by separate cams driven by the same motor. Incorporated between the motor and the three cams is a variable gear box; therefore the frequency

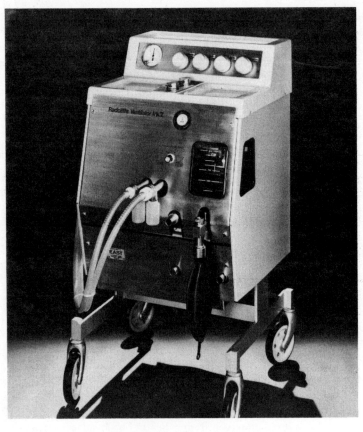

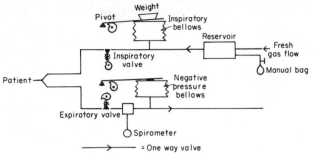

Fig. 10.4. The East Radcliffe Mark V ventilator. This features an autoclavable patient circuit and an infinitely variable respiratory rate control. The ventilator can be used either as a time- or pressure-cycled machine.

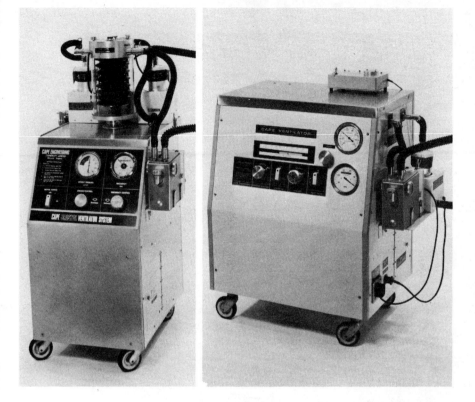

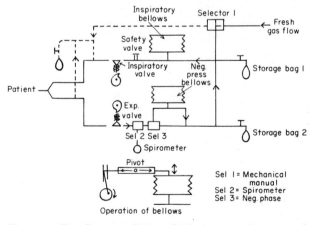

Fig. 10.5. The Cape ventilators. Both these ventilators are fitted with a high efficiency bacterial filter system which protects both the inspired and expired parts of the breathing circuit. This safeguards patients from inspired infection and nursing staff from inherent dangers of expired infections. The Cape Bristol ventilator (*left*) has an additional benefit of an autoclavable patient circuit. The lower diagram describes the right-hand multi-purpose ventilator.

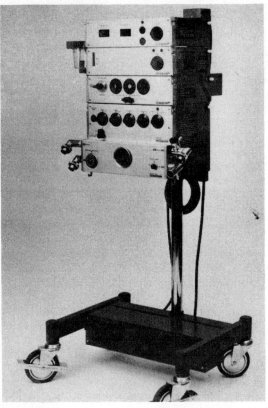

Fig. 10.6 (a) A new electronically controlled flow-cycled Engström ventilator. It has great flexibility and requires a pressurized gas source.

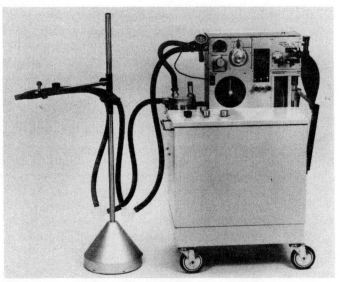

Fig. 10.6 (b) Engström ER300 Series.

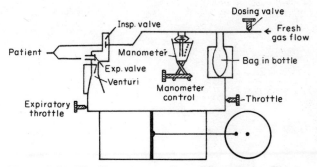

Fig. 10.6 (b). The Engström ventilator ER300 Series. This is a time-cycled, volume preset ventilator. This model has a removable patient circuit which can be removed and sterilized.

of ventilation can be altered although the inspiratory–expiratory ratio remains fixed. Another arm from the gear box raises an expiratory bellows and so a negative phase during expiration can be used. Because of its mode of function this machine cannot be triggered by the patient.

The Engström ventilator ER300 Series (Fig. 10.6)

In simple functional terms this ventilator acts as a flow generator and is time cycled and volume preset. The power supply is electricity which drives a very powerful motor which in turn moves a piston to and fro through an enclosed cylinder. The flow of gas from this cylinder is led into a glass cylinder which contains a reservoir bag. The bag is thus compressed and its contents flow through a non-return valve to the patient. As the piston returns to its former position a negative pressure is created within the cylinder and this is transmitted to the reservoir bag which then draws in gas from either a pressurized gas source or from entrained air. The change from inspiration to expiration is achieved by the opening of a port by the connecting rod of the piston, and so pressure developed within the driving cylinder, which is related to the traverse of the piston, falls to atmospheric pressure. The machine is thus time cycled and again there is a fixed *I/E* ratio but the frequency can be changed by altering a variable gear box between the motor and the piston. There is no triggering device but there is facility for a negative phase during expiration.

If *the electricity supply fails* and there is no available pressurized gas source the cams may still be turned manually with a handle provided for this purpose with the East Radcliffe and Cape ventilators. In the case of the Engström a pressurized gas source must be available. However, with the advent of self-inflating bags, i.e. the Ambu assembly, this is not as important as it was previously.

The Blease pulmoflator (Fig. 10.7)

This versatile ventilator may be described in a number of ways. Simply, it is a constant-flow generator which is pressure cycled, but because of the

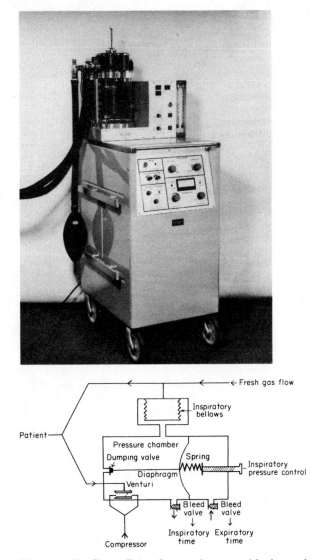

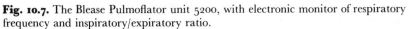

Fig. 10.7. The Blease Pulmoflator unit 5200, with electronic monitor of respiratory frequency and inspiratory/expiratory ratio.

reserve of power within the machine it can also be used as a volume-preset machine and both the inspiratory and expiratory times can be controlled by 'bleeding' the flow from the motor and also by adjusting the sensitivity of the pressure control valve. The power source is again electricity and this drives a large compressor. The flow from the compressor is led into two chambers, one containing a reservoir bellows which empties gas into the patient and another chamber in which there is a diaphragm which allows both chambers to return to atmospheric pressure at a preset pressure value.

In addition to this there is a 'bleed' to the atmosphere interposed between the compressor and the two chambers. If this bleed is closed and the preset level at which the pressure in the two chambers drops is set at a very high value then the volume of gas delivered to the patient can be adjusted by altering the traverse of the inflating bellows.

A venturi system can provide either a negative or positive phase during expiration. There is a triggering device which alters the position of the diaphragm in the second chamber but it is arguable whether triggering is necessary at all. Again there is provision for manual ventilation only if there is a source of pressurized gas.

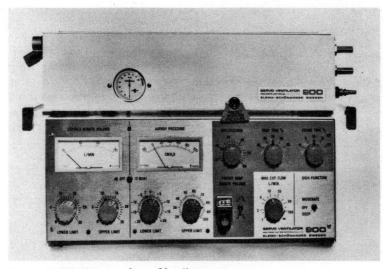

Fig. 10.8. The Siemens Servo Ventilator 900.

Siemens Servo Ventilator 900 (Fig. 10.8)

The Servo Ventilator 900 is an electronically controlled lung ventilator for intensive care and anaesthesia. It can be set for volume-generated or pressure-generated ventilation; controlled or assisted.

Its great flexibility makes it suitable for ventilation of all patients: adults, children and newborn infants.

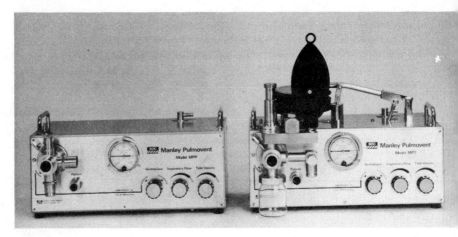

Model MPP automatic

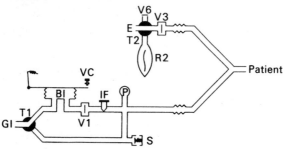

Model MPP manual

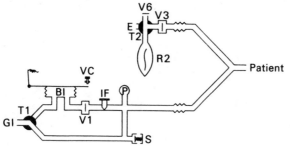

Fig. 10.9. The B.O.C. Manley Pulmovent, models MPP and MPT.

BI	inspiratory bellows	T1	auto–manual tap
E	exhaust	T2	auto–manual tap (patient circuit)
GI	gas inlet	VC	tidal volume control
IF	inspiratory flow control	V1	inspiratory valve
P	pressure gauge	V3	expiratory valve
R2	manual rebreathing bag	V6	manual Heidbrink valve
S	safety valve		

The Manley pulmovent (Fig. 10.9)

This ventilator is a minute volume divider; in other words, regardless of all other parameters it will deliver to the patient the volume of gas supplied to it each minute. It is a constant-flow generator and is volume cycled. The power source is the compressed respirable gas at 7–105 p.s.i. (50–700 kPa), the flow being controlled with flowmeters. This flows into the inspiratory bellows, raising the spring-loaded arm until the volume selected on the tidal volume control is reached. This then opens the inspiratory valve and closes the expiratory valve, and the contents of the bellows empties into the patient via the inspiratory flow control. The end of inspiration occurs when the bellows is then filled again during the expiratory phase by the fresh gas. Expiration is passive in Model MPP but may be assisted by an expiratory bellows which is drawn out by the expanding inspiratory bellows on Model MPT.

References

Hunter, A. R. (1961). The classification of respirators. *Anaesthesia* **16**, 231.

Mapleson, W. W. (1962). The effect of changes of lung characteristics on the functioning of automatic ventilators. *Anaesthesia* **17**, 300.

Robinson, J. S. (1974). In: *Scientific Foundations of Anaesthesia*, 2nd edn., p. 469. Ed. by C. F. Scurr and S. A. Feldman. Heinemann Medical, London.

Chapter 11

Management of Artificial Ventilation

While patients are receiving artificial ventilation it is essential not to become so engrossed with ventilation that one fails to look after the patient as a whole. It is common for those patients who need ventilation to be seriously incapacitated either as a result of concomitant disease of other organs or as a secondary effect following respiratory failure, or they may be semi-comatose or unconscious with cardiac or renal failure. Thus equal attention must be paid to all systems of the body as any malfunction may jeopardize the patient's life.

The long-term management of ventilation also involves the management of a tracheostomy. Orotracheal intubation may be instigated as a short-term measure, but if ventilation is necessary for more than two or three days a tracheostomy or naso-bracheal intubation is usually performed.

A tracheostomy is preferred for the following reasons:

1. Management of the airway is easier because:
   bronchial suction ⎫
   humidification ⎬ are all performed more efficiently
   tracheal toilet ⎭
2. Maintenance of the airway is easier because:
   the tube is shorter
   access is easier
   the tube is tolerated more readily
   it is less irritant
   it is less traumatic
   it is easily replaced
   it is easily cleaned

In addition, blockage is less likely to occur, and is more readily detected, with a tracheostomy tube as opposed to a long endotracheal tube.

Preparation

Given adequate warning, the staff of the receiving unit (respiratory or intensive care unit) must make sure that everything is available to receive the patient. A clean ventilator should be ready for the patient and, from the provisional diagnosis of the patient's pathology, it is important that the type of machine selected should have the versatility and characteristics necessary for the management of that particular patient.

Choice of ventilator

The majority of patients can be ventilated satisfactorily using a machine which behaves as a pressure generator. Those with changing compliance or high airways resistance are better ventilated using a flow generator. Although there has been considerable discussion about ideal pressure waveforms and inspiratory–expiratory time ratios, the theoretical advantages are not always so apparent in practice. Factors which promote satisfactory gas exchange tend to have adverse cardiovascular effects and vice versa. When choosing a ventilator considerations such as cost, reliability, simplicity in use, and ease of sterilization are more important than the pursuit of some pedantic ideal.

Many ventilators are still fitted with a means of applying subatmospheric pressure during expiration though this facility is little used nowadays. Much more important is the provision of positive end-expiratory pressure (PEEP). This technique often allows a lower inspired oxygen concentration to achieve satisfactory arterial partial pressures of oxygen (Pa_{O_2}).

Most adults can be ventilated satisfactorily with a frequency of 10–16 times a minute and tidal volumes of 500–1 200 ml. Some patients feel uncomfortable and fail to synchronize with the ventilator unless large tidal volumes are used. To avoid excessive reduction in the arterial partial pressure of carbon dioxide (Pa_{CO_2}), 'artificial dead spaces' consisting of tubes of internal volume 50–150 ml can be placed between the ventilator tubing and the patient.

In addition to considering the type of ventilator to be used, arrangement should be made for the provision of oxygen enrichment to the inspired gases and a method of humidification. If humidification involves the use of a heated water bath, it should be filled and heated to the correct temperature. Lastly, the ventilator should be tested for (1) residual disinfectant, and (2) gas leaks.

Whenever a new patient is received into the intensive care unit, endotracheal intubation equipment and a good light should be at hand together with adequate suction equipment.

A trolley should be available so that an intravenous drip or a central venous pressure cannula may be inserted if required, and an arterial puncture performed should this be considered necessary. It is preferable to have an intravenous infusion in all patients for the initial phase of their treatment as this will enable the staff in charge to have an intravenous portal for drug and fluid administration and to obtain blood samples for electrolyte, haemoglobin measurements.

A means of measuring the tidal and minute volumes must be at hand and probably the most useful instrument is the Wright respirometer (Fig. 11.1).

A means of manual ventilation must be available, not only for transporting the patient to the unit but also for use if the ventilator fails. This may be a simple apparatus such as an oxygen cylinder together with a bag and mask or an endotracheal adaptor. Alternatively, a self-inflating bag may be used (i.e. the Ambu resuscitator or Laerdal bag) (Fig. 11.2).

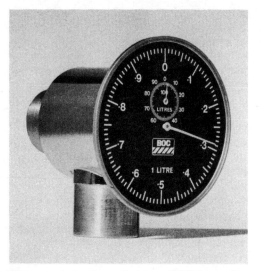

Fig. 11.1. A simple respirometer (Wright respirometer: British Oxygen Company).

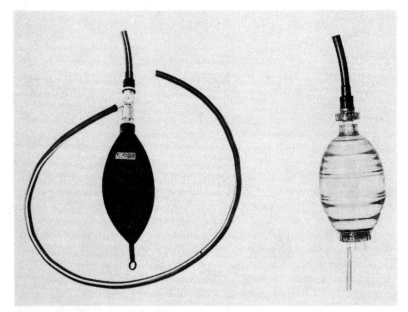

Fig. 11.2. A rebreathing system for high inspired oxygen administration (Mapleson B circuit). On the right is a Laerdal self-inflating bag with a non-return valve between the bag and the patient. Oxygen can be administered into the bag as illustrated. Both these arrangements can be used for producing an artificial sigh and cough during active physiotherapy.

In some units a mobile ventilator is used to transport desperately ill patients (Fig. 11.3).

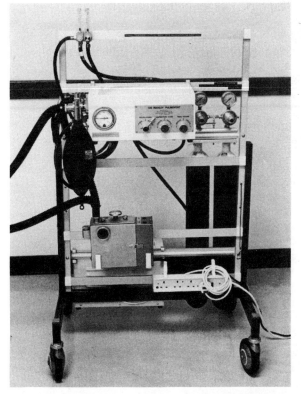

Fig. 11.3. A mobile resuscitation trolley. Here air and oxygen may be premixed before delivery to the Manley ventilator. Compressed air sources may be wall fitments or from the compressor at the base of the trolley. Oxygen may be supplied either from piped supplies or from the cylinders on the trolley. A plug board is also provided at the base of the trolley for cardiovascular monitoring, etc.

Control of ventilation

The ventilator must be set so that it produces an alveolar ventilation sufficient to maintain the blood oxygen and carbon dioxide tensions within a physiologically acceptable range. A suitable rate of ventilation should be selected and the tidal volume increased until adequate ventilation is achieved.

1. Setting the time controls

The frequency of ventilation should be set for adults at between 10 and 16 times a minute and for children at a slightly faster rate. It has been shown that large volumes given at slow rates produce a more even distribution and less increase in dead space than when small volumes are given at a fast rate. Neonates have a normal rate of between 30 and 40 breaths a minute. It is not necessary to provide this frequency when ventilating a child in this age group, indeed it may be disadvantageous to do so. Both distribution and diffusion of the inspired gases take time and so an increase in rate reduces the effectiveness of alveolar ventilation. The relative durations of inspiration and expiration are of vital importance. Inspiration should occupy as short a time as possible, but an adequate tidal volume will only enter the lungs and be effectively distributed to the ventilatory system of the alveoli if given an adequate time to do so. It has been shown that an inspiratory time of less than 1 second results in a decreased ventilatory exchange, probably due to insufficient time for mixing of gas and exchange between inspired and alveolar gases.

In adults the ideal inspiratory time lies between 1·0 and 1·5 seconds. Expiration is predominantly passive and the expiratory time (including both expiration and the postexpiratory pause) should be at least twice as long as the time for inspiration. Prolonged expiratory times may be necessary in patients with severely diseased lungs, especially in those in whom elastic recoil is limited as a result of emphysema. It is interesting to note that in these patients the lungs are relatively expanded in the resting, preinspiratory state, so that elastic recoil is as effective as possible. A very short expiratory period will result in a rise in the mean intrathoracic pressure, with possible adverse cardiovascular effects.

2. Setting the tidal volume

The tidal volume necessary for a particular patient may be assessed in a number of ways. The obvious clinical method is to observe chest wall excursion and when this appears normal the tidal volume delivered is probably adequate. This should then be checked by measuring the exhaled tidal volume and, ultimately, minute volume using a respirometer.

While the Radford nomogram (see Fig. 4.1) gives an accurate basal tidal volume, another rough and ready assessment is to take the weight in pounds as millilitres of dead space and multiply this number by three; this gives a coarse guide of tidal volume:

$$\text{Weight (lb)} \times 3 = \text{Dead space (ml)} \times 3 = \text{Tidal volume}$$

This figure should be increased by 10% when the dead space is increased by positive pressure ventilation.

After ventilating the patient for up to half an hour, arterial blood gases are measured; this, together with another measurement of blood gases perhaps an hour later, allows the adequacy of ventilation to be assessed.

3. Airway pressure

It is often useful, and indeed in small children very necessary, to measure both the tidal volume and the inflation pressure. Assuming chest wall compliance and lung compliance to be normal, a satisfactory tidal volume will necessitate an inflation pressure of 8–10 cm H_2O (0·8–1·0 kPa). Compliance is the inverse of elasticity and is the volume required to produce a unit change in pressure. The inflation pressure in the airway during inspiration together with the tidal volume measured in the expiratory limb of the machine will give the clinician a relative value of the chest wall and the lung compliance (Sykes, 1974).

It is important to record the airway pressure at regular intervals, as any variation will reflect a change in compliance, and therefore a change in pulmonary characteristics. This may be due to various factors such as an alteration in the degree of muscular paralysis or central sedation, the presence of sputum in the airways or the development of pulmonary oedema.

4. Humidification

All patients ventilated for longer than half an hour should be inflated by gases passed through a humidifier incorporated in the patient's circuit. Ideally the inspired gas should reach the patient's trachea with a relative humidity of 100% at 34° C.

5. Oxygen enrichment and blood gases

Though a small number of patients can be ventilated satisfactorily with air, the majority require some degree of oxygen enrichment. The minimum concentration should be chosen which results in adequate haemoglobin oxygen saturation. This is usually achieved by a Pa_{O_2} of 60–90 mm Hg (8–12 kPa). Facilities for measuring the inspired oxygen concentration (such as a paramagnetic oxygen analyser) are essential and progress can often be assessed by observing changes in alveolar–arterial oxygen difference.

6. Oxygen availability

In a patient with a normal cardiac output and haematocrit the danger of hypoxia is present if the Pa_{O_2} falls below 60 mm Hg (8 kPa), due to the shape of the oxygen dissociation curve; however, in patients with low cardiac output states or anaemia, every effort should be made to keep the Pa_{O_2} as near normal as possible.

Oxygen availability is the amount of oxygen presented to the respiring tissues each minute. Alternatively, this may be expressed as:

$$\frac{\text{Available}}{\text{O}_2/\text{min}} = \left(\frac{\text{Haemoglobin}}{\text{content}} + \text{Plasma content} \right) \times \text{Cardiac output}$$

From this equation it can be seen that the important factors are haemo-globin content, O_2 saturation and cardiac output. The plasma content of oxygen is small and only important in hyperbaric oxygen therapy.

High inspired oxygen levels are sometimes necessary but ventilation for more than a few hours with concentrations above 50% may result in pulmonary oxygen toxicity. It is usually of no benefit to increase the inspired concentration beyond 80% as a high alveolar oxygen tension may cause an increase in pulmonary shunting with paradoxical reduction in Pa_{O_2}. The addition of PEEP is useful for reducing alveolar–arterial oxygen differences and the effect of this manoeuvre should be assessed in any patient in whom an inspired oxygen concentration of 50% fails to maintain adequate arterial oxygenation.

Patients tolerate artificial ventilation more satisfactorily when their Pa_{CO_2} is 5–10 mm Hg (0·7–1·3 kPa) below its usual value. For most patients values of 30–35 mm Hg (4·0–4·7 kPa) are sufficient while for those with severe respiratory disease values of 45–60 mm Hg (6–8 kPa) are acceptable. Greater reductions usually achieve no benefit and may delay the return to spontaneous respiration. A fall in blood pressure is not uncommon during the first hours of artificial ventilation, particularly if the patient was previously hypoxic or hypercarbic. A sudden fall in Pa_{CO_2} and the relief of hypoxia may reduce sympathetic drive sufficiently to cause hypotension.

In some patients the arterial partial pressure of carbon dioxide (Pa_{CO_2}) may be reduced deliberately as a therapeutic measure. Some authorities advocate hyperventilation in cases of acute head injury to reduce intracranial pressure, when a Pa_{CO_2} of 25–30 mm Hg (3·3–4·0 kPa) is recommended.

Blood-gas analysis also includes an estimate of metabolic disturbances of acid–base balance. Any persistent deviation from normal requires investigation. Among the important causes of metabolic acidosis are inadequate peripheral circulation, infection, diabetes and poorly planned intravenous feeding regimens. Potassium depletion is a cause of metabolic alkalosis which is often overlooked.

The ventilatory control of a patient

In order to control the ventilation of a patient efficiently, spontaneous ventilation must be suppressed. This may be done in one of two ways: either by paralysis of the patient's musculature with a long-acting non-depolarizing muscle relaxant such as pancuronium or curare, or by the depression of central respiratory function using analgesics or neuroleptanalgesic mixtures. It is also possible to remove central respiratory drive by hyperventilation, though the effects of hyperventilation on cerebral blood flow and function may make this procedure hazardous. The use of analgesic or neuroleptanalgesic mixtures to remove respiratory drive is the most commonly used method of controlling ventilation, drugs such as droperidol 5–10 mg with phenoperidine 1–2 mg, pethidine 25–50 mg and diazepam 5–10 mg being most commonly used for adult patients of an average size. It is undesirable for the patient to attempt to breathe spontaneously while being ventilated.

'Fighting the ventilator'

This is an attempt by the patient to breathe spontaneously. It can produce excessive positive pressure within the airway, it is wasteful for the patient to make this effort and is likely to lead to inefficient ventilation.

There are two reasons for a patient to 'fight the ventilator':

1. Ventilation may be inadequate to keep the blood-gas levels within the physiological range, resulting in triggering of the hypoxic drive or a direct effect of hypercarbia on the respiratory centre. This may be due to a change in pulmonary characteristics. Secretions may increase and if the machine cannot overcome the obstruction then ventilation will be insufficient. This is very obvious in pulmonary oedema. Alternatively, a pneumothorax may change not only the distribution of pulmonary ventilation but also blood flow and so result in oxygen desaturation.

2. The patient may be recovering from the disease process which caused the ventilatory insufficiency or from drugs given to abolish respiration. If recovery is sufficiently advanced, the patient may be weaned from the ventilator in a progressive and controlled fashion; otherwise, additional sedation may be required.

Recording of parameters

Having established adequate ventilation for the patient, the following measurements must be made at frequent intervals and any gross change in them must be reported to the clinician in charge, as they may have serious import. A suitable record chart must be kept:

1. Frequency of ventilation (pump rate). This should be recorded every 15 minutes.

2. Tidal volume (exhaled from the patient). This should be recorded every 15 minutes.

3. Minute volume (Wright respirometer). Recorded every 15 minutes.

4. Peak airway pressure. This should be measured every 15 minutes.

5. Arterial diastolic and systolic blood pressure—every 15 or 30 minutes.

6. Pulse rate—every 15 or 30 minutes.

7. The temperature of the water in the humidifier, if the hot water reservoir type is used, should be measured every 30 minutes.

In addition, the following observations should be recorded every 6 hours:

1. *Suction.* The quantity and nature of the secretions aspirated during routine suction of tracheostomy and endotracheal tubes should be noted (i.e. mucous, mucopurulent, purulent, serous, blood-stained).

2. *Oxygen flow to the machine.* The flow supplied to the machine does not equal the flow delivered to the patient. The oxygen flow coming to the machine is the number of litres supplied to the machine in each minute, but

the inspiratory bellows will only fill during expiration. During inspiration, although the oxygen is being supplied to the machine, it is not flowing into the inspiratory bellows. If there is a collecting bag on the upstream side of the inspiratory bellows or if the air-oxygen mixture is delivered by a venturi or piped pressurized gases then the nomogram in Fig. 11.4 is of use. The one certain method of assessing inspired oxygen concentration ($F_{I_{O_2}}$) is to

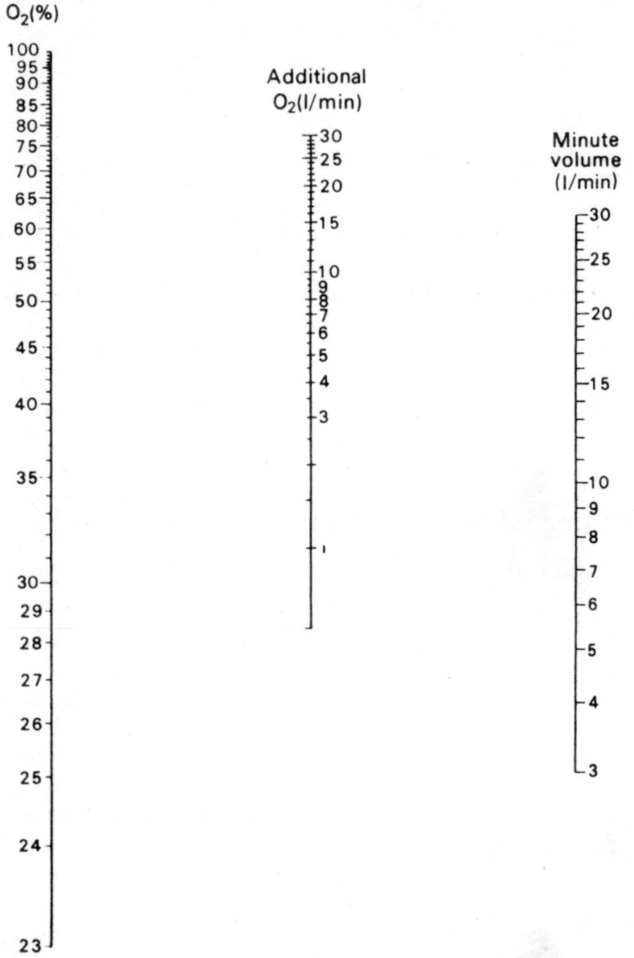

Fig. 11.4. Guide to inspired oxygen. By placing a ruler between the minute volume required and the percentage of oxygen necessary, the additional oxygen (in litres per minute) needed to provide this oxygen level can be predicted.

measure the gas mixture in the inspirating limb as near to the patient as is feasible. A paramagnetic analyser will measure oxygen-air mixtures, and a fuel cell oxygen analyser will measure oxygen in anaesthetic mixtures.

3. *The volume of air needed to inflate the cuff* of the tracheostomy or endo-tracheal tube; this must be noted together with the time and date when the

tracheal tube was changed. It should be borne in mind that the room air will expand in the cuff as it warms up to body temperature. The kind of tube and the size must also be recorded and a replacement must be readily to hand.

It has recently been shown that ventilating a patient with N_2O/O_2 mixtures can result in a dramatic increase in cuff volume. This is due to diffusion of N_2O across the cuff membrane with little or no displacement of N_2 from inside the cuff. It is thus well to remember to inflate the cuff with the inspired gas if anaesthetic gas mixtures are used for longer than half an hour (Stanley et al., 1974).

Management of the patient

In any respiratory unit a doctor must be on call and close at hand at all times. In addition, there should be a daily ward round with all the doctors responsible for the patients. At these meetings the nursing staff should be given instructions which are simple, explicit and direct. Ventilatory and fluid requirements for the day must be decided upon, together with requests for x-rays, urine and blood analysis. Any additives to the fluids given (for example, electrolytes, protein, carbohydrate and antibiotics) must also be recorded. The daily fluid input, including oral feeding, must be itemized and fluid loss assessed, written down and subtracted from the total input.

Thus a fluid balance for the day is fully documented and an adequate intake of calories assured. It must be appreciated that fluid can also be given to the patient in the form of supersaturated inspired gas. The only way to assess the extent of this positive fluid balance is to weigh the patient. Conversely, if the patient is ventilated with dry gases, fluid will be lost.

If a laboratory investigation is to be repeated during the day the time intervals must be given. Ideally all patients should be seen twice a day by the clinician in charge, but all requests must be directed through a final common pathway. Perhaps the best arrangement is for the house physician or surgeon of the unit responsible for the patient to give these decisions to the nursing staff and to write all the instructions and treatment himself. This will prevent a duplication of tests and ensure that the results are available for interpretation by all the doctors responsible for the treatment of that particular patient.

Patient-triggered ventilators

In clinical practice a decision is made either to ventilate the patient or not, and in this context the use of patient triggering has little to offer. However, a patient-triggered ventilator can be useful if the patient has no depression of respiratory drive. When considering the postoperative care following pulmonary resection in a patient with generalized incapacitating pulmonary disease, it is useful to assist the work of ventilation and to reduce oxygen consumption in the postoperative period, although weaning the patient from the ventilator is often difficult. Patient-triggered ventilators may also be useful if the patient has concomitant metabolic disease, or renal dysfunction, as it allows him to adjust the level of respiratory compensation. It may also have a place in weaning patients from ventilators although intermittent mandatory ventilation has largely superseded this technique.

Weaning from the ventilator

In any patient who has been ventilated mechanically for more than about one day the return to spontaneous ventilation is likely to involve a gradual process referred to as **weaning**! There are no hard-and-fast rules for weaning patients from the ventilator but many short periods off the ventilator are generally preferable to a prolonged interruption of mechanical ventilation. A suitable scheme is outlined below.

Initially, and provided that he can exchange an adequate tidal volume without distress and does not become hypoxic and restless, the patient can be removed from the machine for 10 minutes in each hour. Over the course of 12–24 hours the period of spontaneous ventilation is increased until the patient is maintaining an adequate tidal volume over 30 minutes. At the end of this period blood-gas samples are taken, and if successive samples show that the patient is maintaining adequate gaseous exchange then spontaneous ventilation is allowed to continue for a longer period. It is important to note that even though the patient may breathe on his own for many hours, during the first few days it is good practice to ventilate the patient overnight. This prevents exhaustion of both the patient and the staff in charge and allows the safe administration of night sedatives and narcotics.

Before weaning the patient from the ventilator, it is important to make a complete assessment of the total clinical status of the patient because difficulty in establishing spontaneous ventilation may be experienced as a result of malfunction of non-respiratory systems such as renal excretion and hepatic detoxication. Similarly, mild hypoxia and hypercarbia occurring during the weaning period may prove dangerous to a patient with cardiac disease or intracranial pathology.

Certain patients, especially the obese or those with chronic lung disease, may prove difficult to wean using the standard method just described. In such cases Intermittent Mandatory Ventilation (IMV) often proves helpful.

This technique allows the intubated patient to breathe spontaneously between inflations of constant volume provided by the ventilator. The frequency of these 'mandatory ventilations' can be reduced progressively so that spontaneous respiration accounts for an increasing proportion of the minute volume. The mandatory frequency can be increased easily if the patient is to be ventilated overnight or if there is a deterioration in the patient's clinical condition. The additional apparatus required for IMV allows the application of raised airway pressure (analogous to PEEP) during weaning (Downs et al., 1973).

Nutrition

Perhaps the most neglected aspect of caring for the ventilated patient is the maintenance of fluid and calorie intake. The patient must have an adequate protein and fat intake as well as sufficient carbohydrate. In addition, both vitamins and certain mineral salts will be required.

The best method of feeding the patient is to provide an easily ingested semi-fluid diet. If swallowing is difficult a nasogastric tube should be passed, but if there is a gastrointestinal defect preventing absorption of food then the intravenous route should be used.

A reasonable estimate of calorie requirements of a resting adult is about 2 500 calories a day and this can be administered using amino acid, fat and carbohydrate preparations (Black, 1967, 1972).

A guide for intravenous feeding is given elsewhere but some guides for nasogastric feeding are given in Table 11.1.

Infection

Though the problems of infection are considered in detail in Chapter 15, it cannot be stated too often that respiratory infection represents a constant hazard to the ventilated patient. There are many reasons for this. Ventilator tubing and humidifiers can act as reservoirs of infection and nursing procedures conducted without appropriate care can spread infection from the environment to the patient, particularly during tracheal suction. Many patients have their immune response compromised by serious illness and steroid therapy, and the indiscriminate use of antibiotics leads to a selection of resistant organisms.

Tracheostomy and prolonged intubation bypass the normal defence mechanisms of the upper airway and it is becoming increasingly apparent that many infections arise from patients' endogenous flora. The predominant pathogens vary from country to country and from hospital to hospital; in the United Kingdom, Pseudomonas and Klebsiella are the most troublesome at present and anaerobes appear important in aspiration pneumonia.

Positive bacterial culture of the sputum is not an automatic indication for antibiotic treatment. There should be clinical evidence of infection and factors such as nature of the sputum, radiological changes, fever and leucocytosis should also be taken into account.

Psychological care

This important aspect often receives least attention. Patients who are being ventilated need constant reassurance and any procedure must be carefully explained beforehand, especially if it is likely to be painful or uncomfortable. Heavy sedation or apparent coma do not absolve the staff from extending the courtesy and consideration which an awake patient has the right to expect. If possible, the patient should be kept truthfully informed of

TABLE 11.1   THREE EXAMPLES OF PREPARED FOODS WHICH MAY BE GIVEN BY
NASOGASTRIC TUBE

Contents	Amounts	H_2O (ml)	Cal.	N_2 (g)	Ions (mmol/l) Na+	K+	Misc.
I							
Glucose	100 g		400				
Complan	100 g		450	4·9			
Methylcellulose	3 g						
NaCl	1 g						
Vitamins							
$Ca^{++} + Mg^{++}$							
Water + totals	1 000 ml +	1 000	850	4·9	17	28	
II							
Casilan	57 g		256	8·2			
Hycal	1 bottle						
Prosparol	250 ml						
Yoghourt	150 ml						
NaCl	6 g						
KCl	6 g						
Vitamins							
$Ca^{++} + Mg^{++}$							
Water + totals	1 000 ml +	1 000	2 285		102	78	Ca^{++} 680 mg
III							
Milk	1 000 ml		650	5·6			
Eggs (2)	150 g		220	3			
Caloreen	500 g		2 000				
NaCl	2 g						
KCl	3 g						
Vitamins							
$Ca^{++} + Mg^{++}$							
Water + totals	1 000 ml	2 000	2 850	8·6	90	80	

his progress and be told the likely programme for the next few days. False
enthusiasm often leads to disappointment and any set-back should be
discussed frankly.

Anyone attending the patient should be encouraged to talk and chat
even though conversation will necessarily be one-sided. Some patients are
able to communicate easily by using only their lips but for others a writing
pad or chart on which the alphabet and a few simple needs are illustrated
should be provided. Newspapers, television and frequent visits by friends
and relatives help to maintain contact with the outside world.

The use of antidepressants is often suggested, particularly by nurses.
Bouts of depression, weeping and temper tantrums are not uncommon
during artificial ventilation. These episodes are not usually the result of

psychiatric illness but a natural human reaction to the frustration of complete dependence and a realization of the gravity of their underlying condition. The problem usually resolves as the clinical condition improves but in difficult cases the help of a psychiatrist may be sought.

A less obvious indication for antidepressant therapy is the sudden onset of apathy, lethargy and an acute confusional state not explained by hypoxia, hypercarbia or other toxic factors. Such behaviour may be due to an underlying depressive illness and dramatic improvement has been reported following the use of tricyclic antidepressants.

Many studies have shown the importance of maintaining the normal rhythm of day and night for the psychological care of a seriously ill patient. Though hypnotics may be useful it must be remembered that every sleeping tablet carries some penalty in the form of habituation, disturbance of sleep pattern, enzyme induction or drug interaction. Simple measures such as dimming of lights and thoughtful use of side rooms and screens will often suffice.

Cardiac arrest

Because all patients in a respiratory unit are inevitably seriously ill, facilities for the treatment of cardiac arrest should always be available. If the patient is in the final stages of a progressive illness then a previous decision as to the advisability of resuscitation should have been taken.

It is important that the nursing staff recognize cardiac arrest as soon as possible. If the danger of cardiac arrest is considered likely, the ECG should be monitored on an oscilloscope. Both audible and visual warning devices should be functioning. It is advisable to place fracture boards under the mattress of patients in especial danger as this will assist in effecting external cardiac compression should this be required.

If an arrest occurs it is essential that the staff looking after the patient should treat the emergency immediately. If asystole occurs, a sharp blow on the sternum may produce reversal and sinus rhythm. The staff caring for the patient should also be acquainted with the use of the d.c. defibrillator, as ventricular fibrillation is best reversed within a few moments of its recognition. There is no reason why the nursing staff should not perform both these functions. At the same time an alarm system must be at hand in order to summon medical help immediately, whilst continuing to administer artificial ventilation and performing external cardiac massage. A trolley must be available containing drugs, needles, scalpel, rib retractors, forceps, etc. The following drugs are necessary, others are a luxury:

1. Sodium bicarbonate 8·4% (1 mEq/ml or 1 mmol/ml) in 100 ml bottles
2. Isoprenaline, 1 mg in 1 ml
3. Adrenaline, 1 ml of 1 : 1 000
4. Calcium, 10 ml of 10% calcium chloride
5. Lignocaine, 50 mg, 5 ml of 1% solution
6. Digitalis, 0·5 mg digoxin
7. Sodium chloride, 0·9% 20 ml for dilution of drugs

In conclusion, there are three important aspects which must always be taken care of when nursing a patient in this sort of unit; they are respiratory, cardiovascular and metabolic functions. The advice of an anaesthetist, a physician and a biochemist should always be available.

References

Black, D. A. K. (1967). *Essentials of Fluid Balance*, 4th edn. Blackwell Scientific, Oxford.

Downs, J. B., Klein, E. F., Desautels, D., Modell, J. H. and Kirby, R. R. (1973). Intermittent mandatory ventilation: A new approach to weaning patients from mechanical ventilators. *Chest*, **64**, 331.

Leigh, J. M. (1974). In: *Scientific Foundations of Anaesthesia*, 2nd edn., p. 253. Ed. by C. F. Scurr and S. A. Feldman. Heinemann Medical, London.

Robinson, J. S. (1974). In: *Scientific Foundations of Anaesthesia*, 2nd edn., p. 378. Ed. by C. F. Scurr and S. A. Feldman. Heinemann Medical, London.

Stanley, T. H., Kawamura, R. and Graves, C. (1974). Effects of nitrous oxide on volume and pressure of endotracheal tube cuffs. *Anesthesiology*, **41**, 256.

Sykes, M. K. (1974). In: *Scientific Foundations of Anaesthesia*, 2nd edn., p. 220. Ed. by C. F. Scurr and S. A. Feldman. Heinemann Medical, London.

Wretlind, A. (Ed.) (1972). Complete intravenous nutrition. *Nutrition and Metabolism*, **14**, Supplement. Stockholm.

Appendix 1

Nursing care of a ventilated patient

Patient observation

Regardless of whether the patient is being ventilated or not, one of the most important observations a nurse makes about a patient is that the chest circumference is expanding. Both sides of the chest should inflate equally and, if ventilated, in rhythm with the ventilator. The colour of the patient's lips, mucosa and nail beds should be pink and no cyanosis should be visible. His face should not have a look of fear, apprehension or discomfort.

If the patient is being ventilated, lack of synchronization between patient and ventilator needs immediate investigation and treatment. There are many degrees of lack of synchronization, varying from an extra breath taken between each ventilation cycle to patients completely controlling their respiratory rate. Hypoxia, inadequate ventilation, pain, discomfort, fear and a full bladder are some of the causes.

Hypoxaemia

Hypoxaemia is an oxygen saturation of the blood below the accepted normal level. It can be caused by poor pulmonary blood flow or low alveolar oxygen tensions. Low blood-oxygen tension can also be caused by poor diffusion of oxygen at alveolar level. Hypoxaemia is often heralded by confusion, agitation, rising and falling blood pressure and tachycardia.

The commonest cause of hypoxaemia is a blockage of the airways by plugs of mucus; therefore the first line of treatment by the nurse is aspiration of the endotracheal/tracheostomy tube. The patient must also be disconnected from the ventilator and manually ventilated with oxyygen-enriched gases. Reassurance is needed by the patient throughout this procedure. When reconnecting to the ventilator, always check that the oxygen flow is correct and that the tubing is connected. Adequate physiotherapy and frequent suction will often prevent this form of hypoxaemia from occurring.

Inadequate ventilation

When ventilation is inadequate and the Pa_{CO_2} increases, the patient becomes restless and attempts to increase his respiratory rate. Initially the pulse rate and blood pressure will rise but ultimately if the condition is not treated both will drop.

The treatment is to increase the minute volume until the Pa_{CO_2} and pH are normal.

Pain, discomfort

Postoperatively and following major trauma, patients will have pain and discomfort, even the pressure from ventilator tubing or malpositioning of limbs can cause enough discomfort to cause the patient to breathe against the ventilator. Treatment is the use of analgesics, checking machine attachments and the position of the patient.

Fear, anxiety

It has been said that patients cared for by an experienced nurse require less sedation than ones cared for by inexperienced nurses. An unsure nurse can transfer her fears to her patient who can exhibit those fears by breathing against the ventilator. There are many other causes of worry for the patients —their family, their prognosis, the reliability of the equipment, lists but a few. Good communication between the patient and nurse can help to bring those thoughts out into the open.

The underlying cause or causes of agitation must be found before sedation is given to the patient. To use sedation as the first line of treatment is to treat the symptoms and not the cause. If hypoxia is the cause of agitation and sedation is used, it causes the hypoxia to continue and does not relieve the underlying cause of the agitation.

It is probably as important to talk to and reassure an **unresponsive** patient as a conscious one. Even a sedated patient can be put at ease by explanation and calm authority.

Observation of the ventilator

The principles and methods of working of different ventilators has been dealt with separately. Nurses in an intensive therapy unit must understand how the machinery works and know what problems can arise and how to deal with them.

There are some observations which are made continuously:

1. The oxygen flow rate should be stable and the oxygen tubing connected both to the oxygen outlet of the rotameter and to the ventilator.

2. The bellows (if a model is being used where the bellows can be easily seen) is always inflating to the preset amount and fully deflating. This action should be rhythmic and even.

3. The inspiratory and expiratory pressure are at the expected readings.

4. The sounds are unchanged. If the ventilator tubing is disconnected from the patient, the sound will alter and each nurse must be aware of the normal sounds. The sounds will also alter if water collects in the tubing. The ventilator tubing must also be checked for kinking and never supported above the patient's head because condensed water may run into the patient's lungs.

5. Temperature and fluid level in the humidifier.

6. If alarms are attached they should be in working order and switched on at all times.

Record keeping

Records are kept so that the patient's condition and progress can be assessed easily and accurately. The type of charts used will depend upon individual requirements. Although this chapter is concerned with the care of a ventilated patient, the whole patient needs consideration and not just the adequacy of ventilation. The following observations should be considered and recorded where appropriate.

General condition

    Level of consciousness
    Presence of agitation and sweating
    Amount of interest taken in surroundings
    Core temperature
    Dryness, colour and temperature of skin
    Jaundice

Cardiovascular system

    Blood pressure
    Pulse rate and ECG pattern
    Central venous pressure or jugular venous pressure
    Urine output and oedema of hands and feet

Respiratory system

    Blood pressure
    Pulse rate
    Colour
    Assisted ventilation or self-ventilation
    Length of time on or off ventilator
    Amount and type of secretions
    Minute volume
    Tidal volume
    Airway pressure
    Oxygen flow rate
    Level of water in humidifier
    Temperature of water in humidifier

Fluid balance

    Nasogastric fluids and aspirate
    Amount and type of fluids administered
    Urine output
    Drains and wound seepage

Drugs

    Dosage
    Route of administration
    Effect

Nursing care

The planning of nursing care is as important as the carrying out of the care, and this will be discussed later. It is easier to discuss the care under the headings of 'General' and 'Specific'.

General nursing care

Eyes

Half-open eyes can become encrusted or lacerated. They should be bathed in normal saline and have artificial tears instilled every 2 hours. If the eyelids are kept closed these problems are lessened. They can be closed with the use of tapes.

Mouth

Oral intubation can cause increased salivation and, while this aids oral hygiene, one should protect the facial skin from salivary accumulation. Cleaning the teeth with a tooth brush and paste also helps to remove loci of infection and firm positioning of the tube helps to prevent sores and ulcers forming at the mucocutaneous junctions.

Nose

Nasal intubation is much easier for nursing management as well as being more comfortable for the patient but nasal tubes can cause pressure and irritation. The presence of a nasogastric tube in the other nostril increases the risk of septal erosion. If the endotracheal tube is fixed firmly and the nostrils are kept clean, erosion will be avoided.

Limbs

Because lack of movement can result in disuse atrophy and wasting, limbs need passive and active exercises. This is done by the nursing and physiotherapy personnel. There are different schools of thought about methods of exercises but all agree that lack of exercise to the limbs can cause contractions and deformities which can prolong the patient's stay in hospital. Adequate support for dorsiflexion of the feet can also prevent foot drop.

Feeding

Feeding is dealt with in Chapter 12, but the timing of nasogastric or oral feeding is planned so that other events such as physiotherapy or postural drainage are not carried out on a full stomach, causing regurgitation.

Bladder, bowels

An indwelling catheter needs regular cleaning and the collection unit should be changed daily. A patient without an indwelling catheter needs to be offered a bedpan or urinal regularly. Urinalysis is carried out daily and a once or twice weekly specimen is checked bacteriologically. Regular bowel actions are important and the patient may require a small regular enema or aperient.

Fluids

The oral route for feeding and fluid intake is to be preferred but intravenous sites are used for supportive and therapeutic measures and are often the only way of providing fluids and nourishment in patients with an inactive bowel.

The giving sets used for fluid administration are changed after every unit of blood or plasma.

Giving other fluids only requires daily changing of giving sets. Intravenous sites and arterial cannulation sites should be dressed only as necessary. Care should be taken to ensure that no tension is exerted on the cannulae and no undue pressure on the skin from the equipment. Disturbance of the entry site is more likely to induce infection and to dislodge the cannula. Regular resiting of the intravenous cannulae is probably more important.

Pressure areas

Traditionally, pressure areas that require treatment are elbows, knees, sacrum and heels. Patients have other pressure areas which need just as much care and attention:

Tapes securing tracheostomy tube connections between ventilatory tubing and tracheostomy/endotracheal tube
Nasogastric tube
Urinary catheter
Intravenous cannulae

Pressure from this equipment can be prevented by good nursing care.

Specific nursing care

Tracheostomy wound

Postoperatively a tracheostomy needs careful observation for the amount of blood loss. The dressing should be changed only when necessary for the first 24 hours, and thereafter replaced with a dry dressing and changed every 4–6 hours. When changing a tracheostomy dressing a strict aseptic technique is essential to prevent infection. One of the main causes of wound breakdown is copious secretions with or without infection.

The tracheostomy skin area should be cleaned with antiseptic lotion using sterile techniques. The same area and surrounding skin is then dried and painted with a spirit-based antiseptic (e.g. mercurochrome 2%). To protect the skin from wound leakage and tracheal aspirate a single-layer, dry, non-adherent dressing (e.g. Melolin) should be used. Very often after the tracheostomy has been in place for several days, the stoma can be nursed without dressings in order to observe the wound edges and it can be kept dry by sucking excess secretions away with a sterile suction catheter. Mercurochrome protects the skin well and bulky dressings can damage the stoma by lifting the tracheostomy tube out of alignment.

Later, when the patient is able to breathe on his own and tolerate a silver tube, it is important to teach the patient to wipe away excess secretions himself.

Tracheostomy tube

There are many types of tracheostomy tubes available, but for use with artificial ventilation the tube must have an inflatable cuff which will seal the trachea. Overinflation of the cuff will cause tracheal necrosis, while underinflation will allow an air leak making ventilation inefficient and will also allow inhalation of vomit. The presence of a nasogastric tube lying in the oesophagus will increase the risk of the formation of a tracheo–oesophageal fistula.

Tracheostomy tubes are normally changed every fifth or sixth day and, if possible, prior to a week-end since nursing cover in intensive therapy units is always most difficult to maintain at this time. The first tube change should be carried out by a member of the medical team and then, if no difficulty is encountered, any further tube changes can be carried out by trained nursing personnel.

Lungs

Clinically the performance of the lungs can be seen by observing chest expansion, listening to the air entry with a stethoscope and biochemically by measuring blood-gas tensions. Chest x-rays are useful for confirming a diagnosis but should not be performed daily without good reason.

To help lungs function to the best of their ability, any secretions which are collecting in the smaller airways must be removed. This is done by positioning, physiotherapy, including postural drainage and aspiration of secretions.

The patient's position is altered 2-hourly from side to side in order to encourage the lungs to alternately expand well and as a preventive measure for pressure sores. In spinal or chest injuries this procedure may be limited.

Aspiration of secretions

The procedure for aspirating secretions is as follows:
1. Wash hands.
2. Explain procedure to patient.
3. Test suction apparatus is working and set at required level of suction.
4. Unwrap and put on sterile glove.
5. Select catheter, tear off end with ungloved hand.
6. Withdraw catheter from sterile wrapping, using gloved hand (only touch end of catheter to be attached to suction tubing with ungloved hand).

7. Remove cap of Cobbs or Swivel connection on endotracheal/tracheostomy tube.

8. Insert catheter gently until it reaches point of resistance.

9. Connect suction tubing to catheter, withdraw slowly, rotating catheter all the time (unless angled catheter used).

10. Recap tube, check patient's colour and ventilator.

11. Reassure patient.

12. Repeat if necessary, using clean catheter and glove.

13. If pharyngeal suction is also required the same catheter may then be used for this if rinsed through with water or saline first.

N.B. This is a sterile technique and a new catheter and glove should be used each time. Always explain to the patient what you are going to do and reassure them throughout. Never leave the suction tube in longer than you can hold your own breath, as you are obstructing the patient's airway. Never connect suction before withdrawing the catheter as kinking of suction tubing can build up pressure and injure the tracheal mucous membrane. Instillation of normal saline and rebreathing with pure oxygen may be necessary at times but usually only during physiotherapy and not as a regular half-hourly procedure.

When aspirating infants' tubes it is sometimes necessary to lubricate the suction catheter with sterile normal saline before inserting it. This allows easy passage of the catheter down narrow-lumen endotracheal/tracheostomy tubes.

Communication

The most commonly used method of communication is speech. Intubated patients cannot use this method and so other means must be made available:

Pen and paper
Bell
Letters of the alphabet enlarged so that patients who are too shaky to write can point to letters and spell out words
Radio, newspapers, 'talking' books

Apart from the patients experiencing difficulty in communication, their relatives and friends can experience difficulty in talking to them. Nurses can be a great help in educating relatives or just in giving extra support at this time by sitting and chatting with them and the patient.

Experienced nurses can often anticipate the patient's needs, and lip reading and sign language can be easily mastered.

Organization of nursing services

Good nursing care does not mysteriously occur; it happens because of advance planning at ward and bedside levels. Duty rotas are organized so that a balance is maintained between new and experienced staff. New staff are orientated to the geographical layout of the unit and to the nursing care required by the type of patient. Suitable equipment is available and in working order.

The bedside nurse must plan her care according to:

1. Patient's needs
2. Ward routines
3. Doctor's ward rounds
4. Physiotherapist's rounds
5. Radiographers

There are many ways of planning patient care. For new nurses a written plan which is broken down into a timetable can be beneficial but if the nurse is not flexible, can become a hindrance.

The following is an example of a nursing care plan from 07.30–13.00:

07.30 Chat to patient
    Take report from night staff
    Check patient's condition
    Check: Ventilator and humidifier
        Charts
    Fluid totals
    Kardex
    Suction
    Oxygen
    Intubation tray
    Spare tracheostomy tube
    Tracheal dilators

08.00 *Patient Observations/Recording*
    Chest expansion
    Colour
    Blood pressure, pulse, temperature, central venous pressure
    Intravenous fluids given
    Urinary output
    Level of consciousness
    Ventilator Observations/Recordings
    Minute volume
    Tidal volume, respiratory rate
    Airway pressure
    Humidifier: fluid level
         temperature
    Oxygen: flow rate
        tubing connected to flowmeter and ventilator
    Aspirate tracheostomy tube, note amount and type of secretions.

(Compare all these observations with the last ones recorded by night staff and discuss any changes with night nurse.)

09.00 Patient observations and recordings
    Ventilator observations and recordings
    Aspirate tracheostomy tube
    Position patient for chest physiotherapy
    Draw blood for biochemical investigations

09.30 Chest physiotherapy
    Position on back

10.00	Patient observations and recordings
	Ventilator observations and recordings
	Aspirate tracheostomy tube
	Oral hygiene, eye care and pressure areas
	Chest x-ray, then position on left side
	Nasogastric feed
	Drugs
	Tracheostomy dressing
	Check any changes in orders following doctor's ward round
11.00	Patient observations and recordings
	Ventilator observations and recordings
	Aspirate tracheostomy tube
	Leave patient to rest or read mail/newspapers, or chat if patient would prefer
11.30	Write Kardex
	Check all charts are up to date
12.00	Patient observations and recordings
	Ventilator observations and recordings
	Aspirate tracheostomy tube
	Oral hygiene, eye care, pressure areas
	Exercise limbs
	Turn on to right side
12.30	Check equipment
	Tidy bedside area
	Report to afternoon staff

Appendix 2

Physiotherapy care of a ventilated patient

Chest physiotherapy in intensive care and cardiothoracic units

Objectives

1. *To prevent chest complications*

    a. preoperatively

    b. postoperatively

    c. overdose

1. Preoperative breathing exercises: diaphragmatic and lower lateral costal breathing. To teach patient respiratory control
2. Try to improve any underlying lung disease before anaesthetics
3. Familiarize patient with postoperative treatment and gain confidence
4. Demonstrate to patient how to support incision site when necessary

As 1 and 4 above and also

5. Encourage cough (with support of incision site when necessary)
6. Encourage mobility in bed when possible

As 1, 5 and 6

2. *To improve air intake and output* due to the following pathological lung changes:
a. Mechanical obstruction (e.g. mucous plug)

1. Postural drainage
2. Percussion
3. Breathing exercises
4. Teaching an effective cough
5. Humidification, inhalations, fluid intake

    b. Bronchospasm

6. Chemotherapy with Bird IPPB machine with the administration of a bronchodilator (e.g. salbutamol) via the nebulizer. Usual dose 0·5 to 2 ml of salbutamol, depending on other medications, plus 2 ml of sterile normal saline for 10 minutes every 4 hours, or as physician prescribes.
7. Relaxed breathing pattern

    c. Loss of elasticity (e.g. fibrosing alveolitis)

As 1, 2 and 3

d. Chest deformity (e.g. scoliosis)	8. Thoracic mobility exercises
e. Muscle paralysis—when partial or full recovery is expected (e.g. Poliomyelitis)	9. Bird respirator set to gently given resistance to inspiration. This can be increased as respiratory muscles recover power
f. Pain	10. Adequate analgesia prior to treatment. Entonox gas may be used during treatment

---

Techniques of chest physiotherapy

1. Pre and post operation breathing exercises	
a. *Diaphragmatic expansion* and breathing control	Aims to improve air entry into the bases of the lungs. The patient is instructed to relax the abdomen on inspiration and pull in the abdomen on expiration, this lowers and raises the diaphragm on inspiration and expiration respectively
b. *Lower lateral costal expansion:* bilateral or unilateral	Aims as above but the patient's hand or helper's hand is placed against the side of the lower rib cage. The patient concentrates on inspiring air down to where the hand is to get maximal inspiratory movement to this area
2. *Percussion:* clapping, shaking or vibtratory	On the chest wall to dislodge sputum from the bronchi and bronchioles. Care with elderly patients, patients on steroids etc., as the ribs will be osteoporotic and prone to fracture
3. *Rib springing*	Increase of manual pressure on the chest wall on exhalation, small extra pressure at end of exhalation with quick release of pressure at the start of inspiration. Exhalation is deepened with corresponding increase in inhalation. Care as with percussion
4. *Humidification*	
a. Inhalations	e.g. Menthol and tinct. benz. co. inhalations
b. Encourage oral fluid intake	Especially in reluctant and/or confused patients. Hot drinks most effective
c. Swedish nose (vapour-condenser)	Placed in tracheal opening of the Portex tubes
d. Bird	With sterile normal saline in nebulizer

5. Postural drainage	Patient placed in specific position to allow gravity to drain each bronchopulmonary segment. Usually half hour maximum and in conjunction with 1, 2, 3 and 4d above
6. Mobility exercises	For thorax, spine, shoulder movement, especially on incision side of chest
7. Nasopharyngeal suction	When patient is unable to cough effectively enough for expectoration. Often used once to stimulate a stronger cough
	All methods should be selected and adapted for each patient and chest problem to obtain maximum improvement in respiration with minimum distress or exhaustion; e.g. children's breathing exercises are turned into games by blowing bubbles, paper windmills or bits of paper tissues off the palm of the hand

Information needed by physiotherapist or nurse prior to chest treatment in cardiothoracic and intensive care units
1. Read postoperative notes
2. Observe patient's colour
3. Respiratory rate
4. Temperature
5. Pulse rate
6. Blood pressure
7. Recent chest x-rays
8. Chest drain, clamped or unclamped
9. Blood gases results
10. Sputum amount, colour, type, blood-stained or not
11. Adequate analgesics prior to treatment (care, as these can depress respiration)
12. Listen to chest pre and post treatment

Aids to increase effectiveness of treatment

1. Analgesics	*see p. 106.* Entonox gas decreases pain without respiratory depression. Gas can be self-administered
2. Drainage tubes	Unclamped during treatment or when moving patient. Whenever possible do not treat with drain clamped (occasionally have to treat, but *gently* as increase in intrathoracic pressure may cause or increase an air leak)

3. Humidification	*see Techniques, section 4.* Useful to help loosen tenacious sputum at back of throat and eases the soreness after extubation; also eases pain of cough
4. Nasopharyngeal suction	*see Techniques, section 7.* Often once only necessary, to show patient he is capable of effective coughing

Changes in techniques due to the following complications

1. Pulmonary oedema	No treatment until medically under control. Then treatment to assist removing secretions and re-expand lungs
2. Compressions of left main bronchus	Due to grossly enlarged heart, can cause collapse of left lower lobes. Lie patient on (R) side for treatment
3. Pleural effusion	With or without aspiration—expansion exercises to prevent restricted lung movement due to pleural thickening
4. Breakdown of sternal sutures	Self-support or nurse supports suture line on coughing. Entonox use to ease pain. No lateral pressure on chest wall when percussing if chest incision
5. Renal failure and patient on peritoneal dialysis	Treatment best carried out when dialysis just finished and the peritoneum is empty of fluid. Allows basal expansion
6. Hypertension, i.e. after coarctation correction	May not be advisable to lie patient flat. Treatment must be gentle
7. Tenacious sputum in infants	Treatment within humidification tents. Infants' airways block very easily and quickly due to thick secretions

Changes in techniques due to the following complications of surgery

1. Surgical emphysema	Air in the tissues from communication of the lung and pleura. Usually disappears without treatment. Paroxsymal or energetic coughing should be avoided, huffing can be done to rid secretions

2. Sputum retention

Preoperative breathing control aims to eliminate this but when it occurs treat using some or all techniques, adapted to patient's condition

3. Pneumonectomy with partial removal of pericardium

Heart may be embarrassed if patient lies on pneumonectomy side. Treatment in sitting position only until heart rhythm returns to normal

4. 'Sleeve' resection lobectomy

The lower lobe is anastamosed with the main bronchus. Oedema usual at the junction and sputum more difficult to clear. Often bleeding into the lower lobes increases the tenacity of sputum by clotted blood present

5. Injury to recurrent laryngeal nerve

After thyroidectomy and pneomonectomy. Causes inability to close the vocal cords. Coughing power lessened. Treatment with the Bird ventilator if permitted, but inspiratory pressure should be lowered to around 10 cm H_2O (1 kPa)

6. Phrenic nerve damage

In pneumonectomy causes paralysis of one side of the diaphragm with paradoxical movement of one dome on breathing. Bird ventilator helps if permitted

Chapter 12

Parenteral Nutrition

Aspects of the post-traumatic situation

In health there is dynamic equilibrium of body protein. It is constantly being broken down and rebuilt, but the processes are strictly balanced.

After trauma, catabolism is accelerated at a time when there is frequently no significant intake of food. The degree of catabolism correlates closely with the degree of trauma. To all intents and purposes the catabolic phase is obligatory, though it can certainly be modified by the administration of amino acids and energy sources. There is a well known metabolic pattern after injury:

1. A *catabolic phase*, which is customarily measured in grams of negative nitrogen balance. As a broad generalization, uncomplicated major surgery produces negative nitrogen balances of 10–15 g, and complicated major surgery 20 g or more. Severely burnt patients have been shown to have negative N (nitrogen) balances of 50 g/day. The following table gives the generally accepted equivalents:

$$1 \text{ g N} = 25\text{–}30 \text{ g lean tissue}$$
$$6\text{·}25 \text{ g protein}$$
$$.5\text{–}6 \text{ g amino acids}$$

Simple arithmetic shows why patients with major septic complications can easily lose 3 kg of muscle per week.

2. A turning point when a sense of well-being returns.
3. Anabolism lasting around 3–4 weeks.
4. Fat replacement lasting as long as 3–6 months, after serious injury.

If catabolism persists, as may occur after serious burns, massive trauma or abdominal surgery with septic complications for instance, the patient becomes progressively debilitated. Protein malnutrition at this time has been clearly shown to be associated with poor wound healing and/or dehiscence, anastomatic breakdown and diminished resistance to infection. Depletion of liver protein causes a reduction in antibody levels and a fall in serum albumin. In fact, serum albumin bears a considerable proportion of the early catabolic process. The destruction of intracellular contents has other more subtle effects such as the liberation of phosphate and sulphate ions (3–4 mEq fixed acid/g N 1.5–2 mmol/g) and potassium loss

(16–18 mEq/g N or 8–9 mmol/g N). Thus, where there is associated relative or absolute gastrointestinal failure, one should now be able to appreciate the importance of parenteral nutrition.

The major purpose of post-traumatic catabolism is generally agreed to be the provision of carbohydrate intermediates for the injured organism which cannot now obtain food and has depleted its liver glycogen. Glucose is the normal substrate for brain metabolism. In the absence of carbohydrates, ketosis supervenes, but there is interesting new evidence that mild degrees of ketosis are actually beneficial and this work will be described later.

In starvation states (and this virtually applies to the usual postoperative administration of 2 or 3 litres of isotonic dextrose), the rates of breakdown of fats and lean tissues have been shown to be approximately equal, with the fat supplying seven times as many calories as the lean tissue. Note that the fat patient has an identical protein catabolism after trauma.

After injury, highly complex endocrine changes occur. To summarize, there is marked insulin antagonism due to raised levels of adrenaline, glucagon, cortisol and growth hormone (GH). For their specific effects, adrenaline and glucagon promote glycogenolysis, cortisol and glucagon induce the formation of gluconeogenic enzymes and lipolysis is promoted by adrenaline, glucagon and GH. The whole situation is compounded by the fact that there is an increased metabolic rate, of the order of 20–25%, but with major complications this can rise to 100% or more. This is said to be caused initially by raised adrenaline levels, which are particularly enhanced by episodes of acidosis or shock from different causes. Adrenaline increases oxidative phosphorylation, and therefore metabolic rates within cells. This stage may then give way to one of increased thyroid hormone activity as it appears that the levels of unbound T_3 and T_4 are raised shortly after injury and are then available to enter the cells (Johnston, 1973).

Insulin levels are actually reduced at the time of injury but rise after a day or two to levels above the normal range. Insulin is a very complex hormone. It is well known that it promotes the phosphorylation of glucose and its entry into cells, and that it is strongly antilipolytic. Its further actions are the promotion of glycogen formation and its highly anabolic effect of stimulating the uptake of amino acids into cells and their incorporation there into protein.

A group in Boston (Blackburn et al., 1973) have used an entirely new approach to the whole problem of postoperative nutrition with extremely interesting results. The aim is to increase the utilization of body reserves of fat. They have found remarkable reduction in postoperative nitrogen losses (1·3 g as opposed to 8·8 g) when 30–60 g of amino acids were infused instead of the traditional isotonic glucose regimen. With this therapy, plasma insulin levels were reduced as there was no glucose to cause its release. In this new situation there is lipolysis and an elevation of free fatty acids and ketone bodies to levels at which the brain can utilize the latter perfectly satisfactorily. There is, however, a feedback mechanism between the level of ketosis and insulin secretion so that only trivial degrees of acidosis occur (2 mmol).

In summary, there are several factors which reduce catabolism—the provision of nutrients, avoidance of hypoxia, shock or acidotic states. Another interesting phenomenon is that warmth reduces catabolism, presumably by reducing the metabolic expenditure involved in maintaining body temperature. Severely burnt patients with massive evaporative losses benefit particularly from a warm environment.

The constituents of parenteral nutrition

For anabolism to occur, amino acids should be given with adequate energy sources. It is usually said that the optimal ratio is 840 kJ * (or 200 calories) for each gram of nitrogen. Fat emulsions are isotonic, but all other sources have to be hypertonic if they are to supply sufficient nutrition without overloading the patient with fluid.

TABLE 12.1. ENERGY SOURCES

	kJ/g	Cal.
Carbohydrates:		
glucose	17	4
fructose	17	4
sorbitol	17	4
Ethyl alcohol	29	7
Fats:		
soya bean	38	9
cotton seed	38	9

Carbohydrates

There has been considerable controversy about the place of fructose in parenteral nutrition, particularly its role in the genesis of acidotic states. Woods and Alberti (1972) have examined fructose metabolism and explained the mechanisms. In summary, fructose is metabolized to CHO intermediates far faster than its aerobic metabolism to CO_2 and H_2O proceeds, with the result that serum phosphate and liver ATP fall, and lactic acid (a metabolic cul-de-sac) is rapidly formed. According to Allison (1974) in a comprehensive review of the metabolic problems of intensive therapy, the reason for this is that fructose enters the metabolic pathways below any rate-limiting steps (see Fig. 12.1). The conversion of lactate back to pyruate requires good liver function, and in many intensive therapy situations lactic acid may accumulate to a dangerous degree, as in shock and/or hypoxic states, and in unstable diabetes mellitus. Reduced liver function is a common feature of debilitated patients in the intensive therapy

* The introduction of SI units necessitates this method of presentation. 1 kcal = 4·186 joules. In the traditional terminology k was omitted so that 1 Calorie implied 1 kilocalorie.

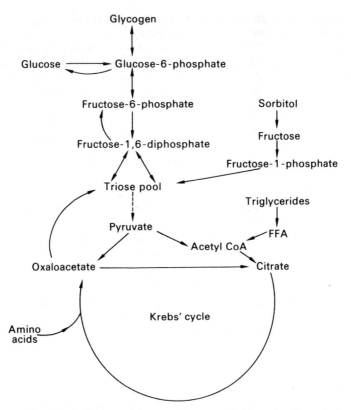

Fig. 12.1. Simplified diagram of intermediary metabolism, showing relationships between glycolysis, gluconeogenesis, the Krebs' cycle, carbohydrates, fats and amino acids. (Reproduced, with permission, from S. P. Allison, 1974, *Brit. J. Hosp. Med.* **11**, 870.)

unit, and is the rule in neonates. Fructose is better avoided in all these situations. In contrast, the initial dehydrogenation of sorbitol to fructose in the liver is rate limiting, and there is some evidence, too, that it is less noxious to peripheral veins.

None the less, the majority of patients can be fed satisfactorily on fructose and it is technically easier. It is not true that the use of fructose avoids the necessity for giving insulin, as large quantities are also converted to glucose.

In the intensive therapy unit the normal substrate, glucose, will usually be the carbohydrate of choice. The rate of intake should not exceed 0·5 g/kg per hour though a faster rate (up to 1·25 g/kg per hour) is permissible in neonates with their higher metabolic rate. The clinician should remember some important points when he chooses glucose:

1. It is not suitable for use in peripheral veins as it rapidly causes thrombophlebitis.

2. Hypoglycaemia, paradoxically, is a real risk especially in small children when glucose infusions are stopped. It is important that it is given at a

constant rate through the 24-hour period. Mechanical pumps or similar devices are usually used in these circumstances.

3. It will almost always be found that insulin is required if the patient is in a catabolic or traumatic state. The administration of insulin has previously involved the use of multiple injections into the patient or the infusion, neither of which is satisfactory, or into bottles of dextrose with the unpredictable adsorption on to glass or plastic. An ingenious method has now been described (Sönksen, 1976) using the precision of a heparin pump, whereby the patient's own plasma proteins can bind the insulin. Frequent checks of blood glucose and serum potassium should be made, especially in the early stages of treatment. Insulin requirements fall rapidly as the catabolic phase is passed.

4. Hypophosphataemia and cellular overhydration have proved a serious hazard in **malnourished patients** receiving hypertonic glucose and synthetic *l*-amino acids (Wright, 1973). The former responded to additional phosphate, but the latter caused far more problems. Normal phosphorylation maintains a low free glucose within the cells, but the unaccustomed administration of glucose/insulin infusions to such patients can swamp the cells with free glucose with ensuing osmotic overhydration.

One must stress that **careless** use of glucose/insulin mixtures with the attendant hazards of hypoglycaemia or osmotic dehydration can be far more dangerous than using fructose.

Ethyl alcohol

This was the first nutritious substance ever given parenterally in the form of intravenous wine administered to animals. The rate of metabolism is such that it can only be used as an adjunct to intravenous feeding, at a maximum rate of 3 litres of a 3·3% solution in any twenty-four hour period. Furthermore, metabolism is dependent on good liver function, it is diuretic, and there are theoretical reasons at least why it should contribute to the formation of lactic acidosis (Woods and Alberti, 1972). The points in its favour are the high calorific value and possibly the pharmacological effect on the central nervous system in a debilitated patient.

Fats

Complete parenteral nutrition is impossible without intravenous fats (or at least essential fatty acids). An intravenous preparation of fat has the advantage of supplying a large quantity of energy in a small volume of fluid which is of neutral pH, isotonic and consequently well tolerated by veins. The calorific value of fat is more than twice that of carbohydrates and fat emulsions provide a very useful intake of phosphate. The fat emulsion is similar to normal chylomicrons. Emulsifying agents are required and the solution rendered isotonic with glycerol or a sugar. Particle size is about 0·5 μm (embolism of small blood vessels occurs at 4 μm). Metabolism proceeds by two methods: hydrolysis by the enzyme lipoprotein lipase, and by the removal of whole particles by the reticuloendothelial system.

There are only two fat preparations available in the UK: one derived from soya beans (Intralipid) and the other from cotton seeds (Lipiphysan). After wide experience over more than 20 years there is no doubt that the more satisfactory preparation is Intralipid, especially where long-term therapy can be anticipated. The recommended rate of administration is 1–3 g fat/kg per day, although far higher doses have been given. For long-term therapy, 2 g/kg should be considered the maximum.

Contraindications to intravenous fat therapy are severe liver damage, coagulation disorders and pathological hyperlipaemia as occurs in diabetics, and in pregnancy as it has been incriminated in promoting the onset of labour.

Protein

The daily requirement of protein for a 70 kg male is 70–100 g. This equates with the commonly quoted figure of 12–15 g of N per day as meeting the daily requirements for an adult.

Blood, plasma and serum albumin are proteinaceous, but none of these agents is useful in parenteral nutrition as a source of nitrogen because the breakdown to individual amino acids is far too slow; for this reason amino acid preparations are used instead. Albumin, however, is largely responsible for the very important colloid osmotic effect of plasma proteins, holding water in the circulation. In some conditions where parenteral nutrition is indicated, albumin or plasma should be given because profuse exudative processes can be expected to occur (burns for instance) and the liver cannot maintain the normal serum albumin level.

Amino acid preparations

The composition of an amino acid preparation is of the utmost importance. It is well known that there are eight essential amino acids and it is important that the ratio of these essential amino acids is balanced, otherwise a reduction in anabolic efficiency will occur. Furthermore, it is apparent that there are semi-essential amino acids. Into the group comes histidine, proline and alanine. Arginine is very necessary in an amino acid mixture, occupying as it does a central position in the urea cycle. Its absence leads to a potentially dangerous rise in the blood ammonia level. It is generally agreed that a preparation supplying all the amino acids is most satisfactory for long-term therapy.

Casein hydrolysate

Aminosol used to be the basis of British practice. There are some limitations to the routine use of Aminosol:

1. A high sodium content of approximately 160 mmol/l, compared with the daily basal requirement of 80–100 mmol.

2. It is an impure preparation pharmacologically: 30% of the preparation consists of incompletely hydrolysed casein. These peptides may on occasion be allergenic.

3. There is a high ammonium content, contraindicating its use in neonates or in patients with hepatic disorders.

On the other hand, milk is a very complete food and the preparation contains very useful **trace elements and phosphates**. It is only with the recent move away from casein hydrolysates that this is more widely appreciated.

Crystalline amino acid mixtures

Body tissues are synthesized from laevo-amino acids. During manufacture both optical isomers will be produced. Racemic mixtures are available (e.g. Trophysan). Dextro-isomers are largely excreted in the urine and can promote an osmotic diuresis. A certain proportion is deaminated and used as a carbohydrate source. Its very high glycine content can cause hyperammonaemia.

Pure laevo-amino acids are available as two different kinds of preparation: those such as Vamin which contain all the amino acids, and others which contain the essential and semi-essential amino acids (Aminoplex, Aminofusin, Travasol, Trophysan-L) with glycine as an inexpensive nonspecific source of nitrogen. Metabolic work is saved by supplying all the amino acids.

The indications for parenteral nutrition
Preoperative

Patients with long-standing inadequate oral intake, severe diarrhoea or malabsorption can greatly benefit from preoperative parenteral nutrition. Note that iatrogenic malnutrition may well be added in hospital while such a patient undergoes recurrent radiological or endoscopic investigation. The patient with upper intestinal malignancy or ulcerative colitis could be expected to show far better anastomotic and wound healing with adequate intravenous feeding, which should start at least 10 days preoperatively.

Postoperative

Patients who cannot be expected to take food orally for many days due to peritonitis or other abdominal trauma, for example, should start parenteral nutrition immediately. Great success has been achieved by many centres treating abdominal fistulae with parenteral nutrition alone. In this way, the flow of bile, pancreatic juice and succus entericus is reduced **below** the fasting level, and the number of organisms greatly reduced.

Increased catabolism

There is a group of conditions where oral feeding may in fact be possible, but intake cannot be expected to approach the metabolic needs of the patient. Such conditions are severe burns, postoperative patients with complications, cases of major trauma and cranial trauma especially where there is increased muscle tone or frank rigidity. Parenteral nutrition is strongly indicated in cases of hypercatabolic renal failure.

Prolonged vomiting or diarrhoea

Included in this group would be conditions such as hyperemesis gravidarum or diarrhoea, which not infrequently follows various tube feeding regimens.

Paediatrics

Newborn infants are being increasingly fed by parenteral regimens. Indications include major gastrointestinal anomalies preventing normal feeding and respiratory distress syndrome; at some centres very low birth weight infants are being successfully fed this way. Remember that the small infant has a far higher metabolic rate than the adult.

Other medical conditions

Patients with respiratory failure and those receiving IPPV often have transitory paralytic ileus. In most major medical illnesses, appetite is usually reduced while energy requirements are increased, although supplementatation can often be given via the gastrointestinal tract.

The above is clearly not a complete list. The **overriding principle** is that parenteral nutrition should be given when oral or nasogastric tube feeding sufficient to meet the metabolic needs cannot be given in the immediately foreseeable future. A major consideration, too, is the danger of pulmonary aspiration associated with oral or tube feeding, in the patient who is dyspnoeic or who has a reduced level of consciousness.

An early resort to intravenous feeding should be made in those patients who have both a highly catabolic state and no chance of immediate gastrointestinal absorption.

Practical considerations and design of a diet

There is no intravenous diet available which can be expected to be satisfactory in every situation. In order to design a suitable regimen certain basic information is essential, including the patient's weight, the renal and hepatic functions, serum electrolytes, proteins, haematological and acid–base status as well as the current fluid balance situation.

A very fair calculation of the daily rate of catabolism can be made from the estimation of the 24-hour urine urea, the change in blood urea and the body weight:

1. Measure urine urea (X) in g/24 hours
$$X \times 28/60 \times 6/5 = X \times 0.56 \text{ (g)} \qquad \text{(a)}$$
(28/60 is the proportion of nitrogen in the urea molecule). If casein hydrolysate is used, the factor 6/5 becomes 4/3, and (1) becomes $X \times 0.62$

2. Measure proteinuria (Y), if any, in g/24 hours
$$Y \times 4/25 = Y \times 0.16 \text{ (g)} \qquad \text{(b)}$$

3. Correct for any change in blood urea, taking into account that body water represents 60% body weight

Rise in blood urea $= Z$ mmol/litre

Change in body urea $= Z \times 60\%$ body weight   mmol

$$\text{Change in N} = \frac{Z \times 60\% \text{ body weight} \times 60 \times 28/60}{1\ 000} \quad \text{g}$$

(molecular weight of urea is 60)
$$= Z \times \text{body weight} \times 0.00168 \text{ g} \qquad \text{(c)}$$
if Z is expressed as mg %, (c) becomes

Change in N $= Z \times$ body weight $\times 0.00028$

4.   (a) + (b) + (c) = nitrogen catabolism in g

(Modified, with permission, from H. A. Lee, 1975a, Intravenous nutrition: why, when and with what? *Annals of Surgery* **56**, 59.)

It is re-emphasized that the patient with major trauma, infection or burns can be expected to have requirements at least double those of the resting state. However, as a generalization, a diet providing approximately 13 000 kJ (3 000 cal) and 15 g of N would be satisfactory in the great majority of ITU cases. Basal requirements are roughly 60% of this figure.

There is an enhanced need for potassium during intravenous feeding, especially when the patient enters the anabolic phase or if the clinician is using the glucose/insulin combination. Assuming normal renal function, 5–10 mmol should be given for each gram of nitrogen. Magnesium is another important intracellular ion and should be standard therapy (0.5–1.0 mmol/g of N). Symptoms of magnesium deficiency resemble hypocalcaemia: tetany and twitchings which may proceed to convulsions and/or psychiatric disturbance. Only Aminofusin contains a realistic magnesium content (every effort should be made to reduce the number of additions to infusion bottles).

Carbohydrates should be given at an even rate throughout the whole 24-hour period as they are necessary for all aspects of metabolism: in this way undue fluctuations of blood glucose are avoided. For high energy regimens a Y-piece system is usually required. In a well planned regimen, fat infusion is begun after the morning blood samples are taken for analysis. The plasma clearance can then be checked, and there is no problem with biochemical analyses. Ideally the clinician should be provided with CHO solutions of several strengths (50%, 30%, 20%, 10%, for instance) so that he can cater for varying fluid requirements (e.g. from anuria to profuse ileostomy loss). Planning is complicated by the various quantities of electrolytes in amino acid solutions. Until one is familiar with the preparations, constant reference to each one will be necessary.

Some suggested diets are given in Table 12.2.

TABLE 12.2.   SPECIMEN INTRAVENOUS FEEDING REGIMENS

Type of regimen	24-hour regimen	Water (ml)	Energy* kJ	cal.	g of N	Comments
Maintenance	1. AminofusinL 600 1 l Sorbitol 30% 1 l	2 000	6 720	1 600	8·8	Extra fluid necessary
	2. Aminoplex 5 1 l 12-hourly	2 000	7 140	1 700	10·0	Very useful for the general surgical ward. Extra fluid necessary
High energy	1. Vamin–glucose 500 ml 8-hourly + Intralipid 20% 12-hourly	2 500	10 900	2 600	14·1	This diet provides 'space' for further fluid, electrolyte or CHO
	2. Glucose 30% 500 ml + 30 mmol KCl 8-hourly + Intralipid 20% 500 ml over 8 hours and Aminosol 10% 1 000 ml over 16 hours	3 000	11 800	2 800	12·8	Insulin and magnesium required. Replace Aminosol with Aminoplex, for example, if sodium content too high

* This presentation *excludes* energy which could be released by catabolic metabolism of amino acids.

The effect of other conditions

In many patients requiring parenteral nutrition there will be pre-existing diseases which necessitate variation in the intravenous diet.

Liver disease

Fat, ethanol and casein hydrolysates are contraindicated. Glucose is the carbohydrate of choice. There may be large, unexpected changes in insulin requirements with changing liver function. The intake of amino acids should be stopped where there is a risk of acute hepatic failure.

Diabetes

In spite of the problems with insulin dosage, glucose remains the most suitable energy source for reasons explained earlier. Fat is relatively contraindicated as there is usually pre-existing hyperlipaemia.

Renal failure

Traditionally a protein-free diet was used in the management of renal failure. However, a diet which contains adequate energy sources and a protein intake of the order of 2·5–6 g N daily is not associated with the catabolic wasting of the earlier regimens and the blood urea rises far more slowly.

In acute renal failure it is often impossible to provide nutrition via the gastrointestinal tract. Full nutrition can be provided with 50% glucose and generous insulin, synthetic *l*-amino acids, fats, vitamins and trace elements. With early recourse to effective dialysis, the abnormalities of lipid and carbohydrate metabolism are seldom encountered. With full nutrition there is frequently a faster recovery of renal function.

Peritoneal dialysis promotes the loss of amino acids and albumin and it is important to provide additional plasma intravenously. The addition of 10 ml of Vamin to each litre of infusate is a useful manoeuvre because it prevents amino acid loss. Fats do not interfere with dialysis membranes. Glucose will be taken up from the dialysis fluid and additional insulin may be required.

The metabolic problems of chronic renal failure are beyond the scope of this chapter. An excellent review of the whole topic has been written by Lee (1975b).

Paediatrics

Fructose (and sorbitol), ethanol, casein hydrolysates and racemic mixtures of amino acids are contraindicated. The formidable technical problems of intravenous feeding in paediatrics have been very well reviewed by Shaw (1973). His technique involves the use of a 19 butterfly needle into the peripheral veins of the arm or scalp. Through this, a fine Silastic catheter is advanced to the superior vena cava or right atrium. Finally a 25 butterfly needle is inserted into the end of the Silastic catheter. (Most workers use glucose, Vamin, Intralipid, dipotassium phosphate, vitamins, calcium gluconate, magnesium sulphate and trace elements.)

Short-term therapy

The use of low-dose amino acid infusions (Blackburn et al., 1973) with far greater utilization of body reserves of fat has yet to pass the test of time;

initial trials are very promising. It is not suitable for the malnourished or diabetic patient.

When nutrition is not likely to be necessary for more than 4 or 5 days the use of peripheral veins is advisable. A new vein should be cannulated daily and this can be conveniently performed at the same time as taking routine morning blood samples. Intralipid will help to reduce thrombophlebitis. If a cutdown is performed, ligation of the vein is inadvisable.

Long-term therapy

Success with long-term therapy depends on obsessional attention to detail with regard to catheter care. Central venous catheterization is essential. Inferior vena caval catheterization is not suitable as it is associated with a high incidence of thromboembolism which is frequently septic.

Superior vena caval catheterization may be achieved via the basilic vein, the subclavian vein, either via the infraclavicular or supraclavicular approach, or via the external or internal jugular vein.

When very long term therapy is likely to be required, infraclavicular subclavian puncture is often chosen. Cutdown on the cephalic vein in the groove between deltoid and pectoralis major has the same advantages and avoids most of the hazards of the blind subclavian approach. Unfortunately, the vein is absent in 5 per cent of normal individuals. The use of these sites frees the arms and neck from strapping and other restrictions. It is an easy area both to keep clean and to secure the catheter. Furthermore, there is a relatively long distance from skin to the circulation, and one needs to leave only a small intravascular foreign body as compared to many other approaches. All these aspects minimize the danger of colonization of the catheter with organisms. After failure to cannulate a subclavian on one side it is essential that the other side be left alone for 24 hours because of the possible hazard of inducing bilateral pneumothoraces.

After insertion, the catheter must be firmly secured, preferably by a stitch very near the puncture site, to prevent it slipping to and fro and introducing organisms. The giving set must be attached very securely and a free reflux of blood obtained on lowering the infusion bottle. An occlusive dressing is applied to the puncture site. Only saline or 5% glucose should be given until a chest x-ray is taken to check the position of the tip of the catheter.

As a daily routine, giving sets must be changed, and the occlusive dressing taken down so that the puncture site may be inspected, cleaned and then sprayed with an antiseptic preparation, such as povidone-iodine. The routine use of antibiotic preparation may cause occasional allergy or enhance the likelihood of Candida sepsis. With this degree of care, drips may run for many weeks, although most authorities recommend changing the site of subclavian infusions every 2–4 weeks (Dudrick et al., 1969). On no account should such a catheter be used for anything else, such as giving blood or taking blood samples. Any interference must only increase the chance of colonization with organisms. Obvious infection of the puncture site is an indication for removal of the central venous catheter, as is unexplained fever, when blood cultures should be taken and the catheter tip cultured after removal.

Vitamins and trace elements

Many preparations contain varying amounts of B and C vitamins; however, a patient should be kept in good health using preparations such as Pabrinex or Parentrovite for 2 weeks. Thereafter, the need for a more complete vitamin preparation becomes necessary, when 1 ampoule (10 ml) of Multivitamin Infusion (SAS Scientific Chemicals, London), or Multibionta (Merck) should be given at least every other day. From this time the patient should have twice-weekly injections of vitamin K (menadiol) 10–20 mg and folic acid 5–10 mg. Vitamin B_{12} 1000 micrograms should be given monthly.

Phosphate requirements are becoming much more important with the recent move towards pure *l*-amino acid preparations. Phosphate is not only required for phosphorylations of carbohydrates by ATP; it is necessary, too, for acid–base regulations by the kidney and for 2,3-disphosphoglycerate (2,3-DPG) in the red cell. Hypophosphataemic states are associated with shift to the left of the oxygen dissociation curve, with the implication of poor tissue oxygenation. Sufficient intake of phosphate is provided if the patient is having Intralipid and Aminosol, or it may be provided as dipotassium hydrogen phosphate 7·5 mmol/l. A word of caution: if one is dealing with a hypophosphataemic state, correction with phosphate alone will produce a dangerous drop in serum calcium.

Calcium is vital in small children but is scarcely necessary in adults for some months as long as vitamin D is given, because of the enormous reserves in the body skeleton. Iron can be given as weekly injections of iron-dextran complex 1 ml (providing 50 mg of elemental iron). Zinc is an important constituent of numerous enzyme systems and in many centres is provided separately. Finally, trace elements such as copper, manganese, molybdenum, chromium and iodine are found as contaminants of protein hydrolysate solutions, but can also be provided by many hospital pharmacies. The requirements of all known nutrients have been comprehensively reviewed by Wretlind (1972).

Summary

Malnutrition should not be allowed to occur in our surgical or medical patients. Relative or complete failure of the gastrointestinal tract can be overcome by giving all known nutrients intravenously. With scrupulous attention to detail, excellent over-all health may be maintained for many months, as can normal growth and development.

Unfortunately, some clinicians still withhold parenteral nutrition on grounds of expense. The cost is unimportant if it prevents mortality, and trivial when compared with the cost of long admission punctuated with recurrent episodes of morbidity.

References

Allison, S. P. (1974). Metabolic aspects of intensive care. *Brit. J. Hosp. Med.* **11**, 860.

Blackburn, G. L., Flatt, J. P., Clowes, G. H. A., O'Donnell, T. S. and Hehsle, T. E. (1973). Protein sparing therapy during periods of starvation with sepsis or trauma. *Ann. Surg.* **177**, 588.

Dudrick, S. J., Wilmore, D. W., Vars, H. M. and Rhoads, J. E. (1969). Can i.v. feeding as the sole means of nutrition support growth in the child and restore weight loss in an adult? *Ann. Surg.* **169**, 974.

Johnston, I. D. A. (1973). The metabolic and endocrine response to injury: a review. *Brit. J. Anaesth.* **45**, 252.

Lee, H. A. (1975a). Intravenous nutrition: why, when and with what? *Ann. R. Coll. Surg. Engl.* **56**, 59.

Lee, H. A. (1975b). Nutritional management of acute and chronic renal failure. *Update* **9**, 601.

Shaw, J. C. L. (1973). Parenteral nutrition in the management of sick low birthweight infants. *Pediat. Clin. N. Amer.* **20**, 333.

Sönksen, P. (1976). Carrier solution for low-level intravenous insulin infusion. *Brit. med. J.* **1**, 151.

Tweedle, D. (1975). Intravenous amino-acids. *Brit. J. Hosp. Med.* **13**, 81.

Woods, H. F. and Alberti, K. G. M. M. (1972). Dangers of intravenous fructose. *Lancet* **2**, 1354.

Wretlind, D. A. (1972). Complete intravenous nutrition. Theoretical and experimental background. *Nutrition and Metabolism* **14**, Suppl. 1.

Wright, P. D. (1973). Intravenous feeding. *Lancet* **2**, 1335.

Chapter 13

Artificial Ventilation, Tracheostomy and Prolonged Intubation in Infancy

Artificial ventilation

Intermittent positive pressure ventilation is now used in infants for a wide variety of conditions which directly or indirectly cause respiratory insufficiency. Examples of such conditions are severe apnoeic attacks in premature infants, prolonged effect of drugs (curare), respiratory distress syndrome of the newborn, pulmonary oedema secondary to congenital cardiac failure, pulmonary complications secondary to congenital tracheo-oesophageal fistula and pulmonary infections. As in older children and adults, respiratory insufficiency may be due to inadequate respiratory movements or to pulmonary complications.

The young infant has much less respiratory reserve than older children and adults; for example, his resting oxygen consumption, per unit of body weight, is twice that of the adult: 7 ml/kg per minute compared with 3·5 ml/kg per minute. In addition, it has been shown that the diameters of distal airways remain constant from birth until about 5 years of age and only then increase in size (Hogg et al., 1970). Infants and young children therefore have a high peripheral airways resistance and a greater tendency to airways occlusion than older children.

The need to conserve heat is a major factor in the management of the newborn infant and this is particularly so in patients with respiratory problems. The average newborn infant has about twice the surface for heat loss for each kilogram of tissue compared with the average adult (Cross, 1965). In a cool environment the infant increases his metabolism to maintain his body temperature and this in turn increases his oxygen consumption and minute volume. Therefore, failure to keep warm an infant who is in respiratory distress, may, by increasing the oxygen requirements, result in respiratory insufficiency. The resultant hypoxia will then aggravate the fall in body temperature because the metabolic response to cold will be impaired. Severe hypothermia will lead to depression of respiratory effort.

The importance of conserving heat in the care of ill infants can hardly be overemphasized.

In severe respiratory distress syndrome of the newborn widespread atelectasis is present and the use of a raised airway pressure (continuous positive airway pressure) has produced a very great reduction in mortality (Gregory et al., 1971). The improvement in the atelectasis brought about by the raised airway pressure leads to a rise in Pa_{O_2} which in turn reduces the pulmonary vascular resistance. Lowering the pulmonary vascular resistance results in improved pulmonary perfusion and a decrease in the right-to-left shunt with consequent further improvement in the arterial oxygenation. Details of the application of raised airway pressure are given on page 149.

Essential features of a paediatric ventilator

1. Tidal volume

The tidal volume of an infant weighing 3·5 kg is about 10–30 ml and varies inversely with the respiratory rate. It is essential that the ventilator delivers at least this volume to the patient. The volume indicated by a spirometer placed in the conventional position on the expiratory limb of a circuit does not represent the patient's minute volume. The figure obtained from the spirometer must be corrected to allow for compression of the gas in the patient's circuit. The gas compressed in the circuit on inspiration will re-expand during expiration when the pressure falls and contribute, with the expired gas from the patient, to the reading on the spirometer (Glover, 1965). The size of this compressibility factor is related to the volume of the circuit, the peak inspiratory pressure and the frequency of ventilation. This discrepancy between actual minute volume and spirometer reading is obviously greatest in dealing with infants requiring high inspiratory pressures. For the same reason the volume setting on the ventilator will be greater than the amount the patient receives. Other methods of measuring ventilation in infants will be mentioned later.

2. Power

The power required to ventilate the infant lung will vary considerably. If the lungs are normal a positive pressure of less than 10 cm H_2O (1 kPa) is required. If the lungs have a high airways resistance or low compliance (e.g. in respiratory distress syndrome or cardiac failure), pressures of over 50 cm H_2O (5 kPa) may be necessary. There are patients with varying degrees of lung pathology between these two extremes.

Consequently, in considering the type of ventilator to use in infants it is not sufficient to consider only the ventilatory requirements of the normal infant lung, we must also consider the ventilatory requirements of the diseased infant lung. Some ventilators, classified as pressure generators, vary in the volume they deliver depending on the lung characteristics. Others, classified as flow generators, are less influenced by lung characteristics (Mushin et al., 1969). The latter are therefore more suitable for clinical use in a wide range of respiratory problems.

3. Accurate control of inspired oxygen

It is now well recognized that high percentages of oxygen administered to premature infants may result in blindness due to retrolental fibroplasia. It is recommended that the Pa_{O_2} in the newborn should be kept below 100 mm Hg (13·3 kPa) and maintained between 60 and 80 mm Hg (8 and 10·7 kPa). (Report of the Committee on Fetus and Newborn of the American Academy of Pediatrics, 1971). Ideally the arterial sample for blood-gas measurement should be taken from the radial or temporal arteries. If the sample is taken from the umbilical artery, a lower Pa_{O_2} may be found than in the radial or temporal arteries due to a right-to-left shunt (e.g. in respiratory distress syndrome).

It must be strongly stressed that there should be no hesitation in raising the inspired oxygen concentration as much as is necessary to maintain acceptable arterial oxygen tensions (Cross, 1973; Bolton and Cross, 1974). There will be no resultant danger of retrolental fibroplasia unless the arterial oxygen tension is abnormally high, and the danger of pulmonary damage from the high oxygen concentration is not acute enough to outweigh the serious and immediate consequences of severe oxygen desaturation.

For these reasons it is essential to be able to control accurately the percentage oxygen delivered by a ventilator. In addition, it is essential to check the inspired oxygen concentration regularly with an oxygen analyser. If oxygen-rich mixtures are administered it is also necessary to check the arterial oxygen tension.

4. Humidification

The need for humidification of the inspired gases is dealt with in Chapter 11. This aspect is often overlooked in considering the merits of various ventilators. It is of even greater importance in infants because the inspissation of secretions resulting from the inspiration of dry gas will readily block the narrow airways of the patient and the lumen of the endotracheal or tracheostomy tube. In addition, it has been shown that a relative humidity below 30% has a retarding effect on ciliary motion (Dalhamn, 1956). We should aim at a relative humidity of 70% or more to maintain ciliary activity.

The methods of increasing the water content of the inspired air are also dealt with elsewhere and will only be briefly commented upon here.

Standard humidifier

If the water in the humidifier is kept at about 55°C then all vegetative organisms are killed. This eliminates an important source of proliferation of bacteria. The temperature of the gases falls as they pass along the inspiratory tubing to the patient. The extent to which it falls depends on a number of factors such as the volume of gas per cycle, the length of the tubing between the humidifier and the patient and the ambient temperature. It is desirable to keep the temperature at the patient end of the tubing at approximately 35°C in young infants and 33°C in older children. In young infants humidified gas is a potent factor in maintaining body temperature as the patient does not have to produce water vapour from his respiratory tract and lose heat in so doing.

Compressed air nebulizer

These give a variable droplet size and a high proportion of the droplets may be comparatively large. Droplets greater than 10 μm are deposited in the upper trachea. Recently there has been a tendency to use heated nebulizers as cold droplets depress ciliary activity.

Ultrasonic nebulizer

These are extremely effective provided an artificial airway is in place. If the patient is breathing through his nose then neither ultrasonic nor compressed air nebulizers are effective because the nose filters out the droplets (Wolsdorf et al., 1969). On the other hand, if they are in use on an infant with an endotracheal or tracheostomy tube in place the output must be carefully controlled to avoid overloading the infant's lungs with fluid. In this respect saline is even more dangerous than water and it is therefore recommended that distilled water is used (Modell et al., 1968).

A serious criticism of all nebulizers is the transmission of bacteria to the patient (Chamney, 1969). The nebulizers readily become infected and are difficult to clean and sterilize. The smaller particles are particularly dangerous in this respect as they penetrate deeply into the lungs where pulmonary clearance mechanisms may not be efficient.

Very few machines will have all four features of a paediatric ventilator described above. However, there are several machines which will be capable of meeting the demands of the less difficult paediatric problems.

Management

General principles

It will be evident that continuous nursing supervision is essential in this work. It is widely accepted now that the objective is to maintain the patient's arterial Po_2 and Pco_2 near physiological levels. Some years ago there was a tendency to overventilate patients. Theoretically, the use of a machine which is triggered by the patient's own inspiratory effort would seem attractive in maintaining normal blood gases. In practice, especially in difficult ventilatory problems in small infants breathing rapidly, it can be extremely difficult to achieve satisfactory patient-triggering of the machine and frequently underventilation occurs. The majority of clinicians today in the United Kingdom take complete control of the respiration.

This is sometimes achieved by the use of drugs which depress the patient's respiratory centre, e.g. morphine (0·2 mg/kg), or by drugs which abolish respiratory movements, e.g. curare. However, if one ventilates infants and indeed older children satisfactorily (i.e. the Pa_{O_2} and Pa_{CO_2} are approximately normal) then these drugs are not usually necessary as the patient will follow the cycling of the ventilator and cease making his own efforts.

There are three exceptions to this generalization:

1. If the patient is in pain, for example in the immediate postoperative period, an analgesic such as morphine may be required.

2. If a patient, particularly an infant, is hungry then a feed is required to establish control.

3. If there are large right-to-left shunts resulting in oxygen desaturation such as in respiratory distress syndrome or pneumonia then the ventilator cannot produce normal blood gases and the patient tends to 'fight the ventilator'. In this situation respiratory depressants such as morphine or muscle relaxants such as curare are required.

In general, therefore, satisfactory control of respiration can be achieved without resorting to drugs.

There are three considerable advantages in this approach to management:

1. *Safety.* If the nurse's attention is temporarily diverted elsewhere and the patient becomes disconnected from the ventilator, he will be capable of making spontaneous respiratory efforts.

2. *Clearing of secretions.* On aspiration of the trachea and during physiotherapy the patient makes much better expulsive efforts and thus greatly assists in clearing secretions.

3. *Warning of underventilation.* Should the patient cease to follow the ventilator it is reasonable to assume that he is not being adequately ventilated, until proven otherwise. There may be many reasons for such a situation: secretions in the airway, collapse of a lobe of a lung, pneumothorax, an accidental change in the settings of the ventilator or a fault in the ventilator—all these possibilities should be checked before resorting to drugs.

Management details

Before putting a patient on a ventilator one should first ensure that those factors which hinder the easy mechanical control of respiration (see above) have been eliminated as far as possible.

The details of managing the patient on a ventilator will vary according to the type of ventilator, i.e. time-, pressure- or volume-cycled, as the method of cycling tends to be the dominant factor in the management. If, for example, one uses a machine which is time-cycled then one fixes the rate and proceeds to increase the volume in each cycle until, at the resultant inspiratory pressure applied to the trachea, satisfactory chest wall movement takes place. It will usually be found that the machine 'takes over' the patient's respiration in about two to three minutes.

It is important for safety reasons to begin with small volumes and gradually increase; this minimizes the danger of producing a pneumothorax.

Ventilator rate

Infants in respiratory distress from whatever cause have a very high respiratory rate because it is easier for the infant to increase his rate of respiration than his depth of respiration. It is not necessary in mechanical ventilation to follow this pattern. Rates of ventilation fairly near the physiological range are satisfactory, i.e. from 30 to 40 per minute. This ensures a larger tidal volume with the possibility that the slower rate of ventilation may result in more even distribution of gas especially in diseased lungs. The latter point is unproven but this approach is satisfactory in clinical practice.

Minute volume

It is extremely difficult to study the normal ventilation in the newborn and the difficulties have been stated in some detail by Cross (1965). There are no precise values for the minute ventilation in the newborn and there are probably wide variations from patient to patient. A useful average figure to take is 600 ml as the minute volume with a tidal volume of 15 ml at a respiratory rate of 40/min in an infant weighing 3·5 kg. It must be appreciated that this is a mean figure.

The next difficulty concerns the measurement of the minute volume when the patient is on a ventilator. The errors involved in using a spirometer on the expiratory limb of the circuit have been described earlier. Accurate measurements of tidal and minute volumes can be obtained by using a pneumotachograph which measures flow and this can be integrated with time to measure volume. However, this requires an airtight fit at the endotracheal or tracheostomy tube and this is not advisable in clinical practice for reasons given later. These instruments require careful calibration and are fairly difficult to use in everyday practice.

Finally, the values obtained are only an indirect measurement of the adequacy of ventilation because of possible variations in the ventilation/perfusion ratio. In clinical practice it is more useful to assess the patient's colour and the adequacy of movement of the chest wall as one would during anaesthesia. The adequacy of ventilation can then be confirmed by blood-gas analysis; a capillary sample from a heel prick is satisfactory except for the Pa_{O_2}, provided the peripheral circulation is good. If the peripheral circulation is poor a peripheral arterial sample should be taken if an umbilical artery is not available.

Pressure

The pressure required to ventilate the lung will depend on the total pulmonary resistance and on the compliance of the lung and chest wall. In the normal infant lung, pressures of less than 10 cm H_2O (1 kPa) are quite adequate whereas in severe respiratory distress syndrome or lung infection, pressures of the order of 60 cm H_2O (6 kPa) may be required.

The correct pressure in a particular patient is the pressure which will produce adequate tidal volumes. The high pressures referred to are not unduly dangerous, provided they are necessary, because the pressure is largely dissipated in overcoming the high airway resistance. They would of course be dangerous if applied directly to the alveoli of a normal lung because of the likelihood of producing a pneumothorax.

Continuous positive airway pressure (CPAP)

This form of support is used most frequently in severe respiratory distress syndrome (RDS) but may also be used in other conditions where there is a tendency to atelactasis. If the infant is capable of regular respiratory movements, intubation is usually performed and an Ayre's T-piece circuit set up. A resistance which can be varied, such as a gate-clip, is added to the expiratory limb of the T-piece. During expiration the patient's airway pressure can therefore be kept at the desired level. Initially, quite high pressures may be required—Gregory (Gregory et al., 1971) used a maximum of 14 cm H_2O (1·4 kPa) in severe cases of RDS—but other workers have used lower pressures.

As the patient's condition improves, shown by the arterial oxygen tension, the resistance is gradually lowered to zero. For the reasons given (pages 14, 143), CPAP also enables lower inspired oxygen concentrations to be used and as improvement occurs the inspired oxygen concentration is gradually reduced. The inspired oxygen-enriched mixture must, of course, be humidified.

To avoid the problems of prolonged intubation in premature infants, Gregory also applied CPAP by using a pressurized headbox with a seal applied around the neck (Gregory et al., 1971). In practice this has not been an easy method and CPAP or mechanical ventilation using a very small facemask have been described from other centres (Allen et al., 1975).

If the infant has prolonged apnoeic spells as in severe RDS then ventilatory support is required. An end-expiratory pressure can then be applied by the ventilator to achieve the same objective as on the T-piece circuit. This is usually referred to as positive end-expiratory pressure (PEEP).

Discontinuing mechanical ventilation

Provided the respiratory insufficiency which has created the need for mechanical ventilation is no longer present, there is generally no difficulty in discontinuing ventilatory support. Where there is some tendency to atelectasis as in RDS or after cardiopulmonary bypass procedures, CPAP using the T-piece circuit is useful before progressing to spontaneous ventilation and extubation. If the ventilator has the facility to allow the patient to breathe spontaneously while the machine cycles at a very slow rate (mandatory intermittent ventilation) this can also be used as a step towards discontinuing mechanical ventilation.

A patient who is unable to tolerate near-normal inspired oxygen tensions is not usually well enough for ventilatory support to be discontinued.

Complications

Most complications and the means of minimizing them have been dealt with already in this chapter. If a pneumothorax occurs, and this ought to be uncommon if correct pressures are used, a chest drain connected to an underwater seal should be inserted and positive pressure ventilation continued.

To avoid the danger of cross-infection the patient circuit ought to be sterilized after being used.

Prolonged endotracheal intubation and tracheostomy

The role of tracheostomy and prolonged endotracheal intubation in the management of respiratory insufficiency has aroused considerable debate since 1962 and many papers have been published on the subject.

Originally, the main indication for tracheostomy in adults and children was upper airway obstruction and the modern era of tracheostomy began when it was shown to be valuable in enabling secretions to be cleared from the respiratory tract in bulbar poliomyelitis (Galloway, 1943). The Scandinavian poliomyelitis epidemics of 1950–1953 led to an extension of this application in order to enable intermittent positive pressure ventilation to be carried out.

This approach to the management of respiratory insufficiency due to poliomyelitis was so successful that it was extended to other respiratory problems in adults and subsequently in infants and children (Swensson, 1962; Aberdeen, 1965; Glover, 1965).

However, some centres had serious and frequent complications following tracheostomy, especially in infants, and alternative methods of providing an artificial airway were sought.

Prolonged endotracheal intubation

Rubber tubes had been used for prolonged intubation but were abandoned for this purpose as laryngeal oedema usually occurred after 24–48 hours' intubation.

The first reported successful use of vinyl plastic endotracheal tubes as an alternative to tracheostomy was made by Brandstater (1962). His series was comprised of 12 children, 9 of whom were under 1 year of age. The endotracheal tubes were in place for periods varying from 3 days to 7 weeks. Of the 12 patients, 9 survived and no permanent damage was seen. However, Brandstater pointed out that he had not performed follow-up laryngoscopies.

This report aroused considerable interest throughout the world and soon reports of larger series from several major paediatric centres appeared (Allen and Steven, 1965; McDonald and Stocks, 1965; Jackson Rees and Owen-Thomas, 1966). These early papers, while pointing out certain complications, particularly subglottic stenosis, were enthusiastic. Subsequent papers (Abbott, 1968o Hatch, 1968) were somewhat less enthusiastic. The latter papers in particular emphasized the serious danger of subglottic stenosis, severe degrees of which result in a very long-term tracheostomy.

Guess and Stetson (1968) identified a factor which may be of importance in causing irritation of the larynx and trachea. They found that slivers of polyvinyl chloride from some endotracheal tubes caused a toxic reaction when implanted in rabbit muscle. The toxic substance was identified as an organotin compound used as a stabilizer in the plastic. This substance has now been eliminated by the manufacturers from plastic endotracheal tubes.

Management and complications

Nasotracheal intubation is used more frequently than oral intubation. Nasal tubes are more easily fixed to the face and there is therefore less danger of ventilator tubing dislodging the tube.

Every complication of an artificial airway (endotracheal or tracheostomy tube) must be regarded as serious and therefore attention to the following details is of the utmost importance in this work.

Incorrect length of endotracheal tube

The length of the tube must be determined precisely because the head may be flexed or extended in the ward, thereby moving the endotracheal tube up and down the trachea. One therefore runs the risk of endobronchial intubation or dislodgment of the tube from the trachea. The only reliable method of determining the length is to measure the tube on the individual patient and not rely on general guides. It is better to err towards the tube being too long because of the serious consequences of a short tube being dislodged.

Kinking

Anaesthetists are very familiar with the danger of kinking in the naso- or oropharynx. With prolonged intubation there is an additional site at which kinking has caused fatalities. It tends to occur where a redundant length of tube protrudes from the nostril and the comparatively heavy connections to a ventilator may readily cause the tube to kink. This is another reason for ensuring that the tube is the correct length.

Erosion of ala or septum of nose

This is caused by the tube, especially if it is distended by a connector in it, pressing on the edge of the nostril. Erosion may appear within 24 hours. If the pressure is not relieved it can cause erosion through the lateral wall or the septum of the nose in a few days. It is very difficult to avoid this complication and Figs. 13.1 and 13.2 illustrate two designs to minimize it.

Figure 13.1 (the Jackson Rees tube) avoids the need for a connector. The inspiratory tubing from the ventilator is connected to one end of the large horizontal tube and the expiratory tubing to the other end. The inspiratory and expiratory tubing of the ventilator is then fixed to the head. While this tube is excellent in the larger sizes, there is a problem in the design which can seriously affect the smaller sizes. This is dealt with more fully below.

Figure 13.2 shows the Tunstall connector inserted in an ordinary plastic

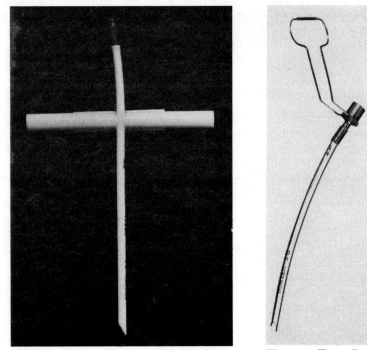

Fig. 13.1. Jackson Rees nasotracheal tube.   **Fig. 13.2.** Tunstall connector in nasotracheal tube.

tube. The main feature here is the strut, the base of which is strapped down on the forehead. By careful positioning of the base on the forehead, the strut pushes the connector away from the anterior edge of the nostril and provides considerable stability so that no undue pressure occurs.

Blockage of the tube

To avoid this complication two conditions must be fulfilled:

    1. There must be excellent humidification for the reasons given earlier.
    2. It must be reasonably easy for the nurse to introduce a suction catheter.

The problem in the design of the Jackson Rees tube referred to above affects the ease of introduction of a suction catheter and is illustrated by Figs. 13.1, 13.3 and 13.4. In Fig. 13.1 it can be seen how the heavy horizontal tube grips the vertical endotracheal tube. In Figs. 13.3 and 13.4 the vertical tube has been cut off at the level of the horizontal tube and the photograph is taken vertically down the lumen of the tube. The protrusions in the lumen of the tube are obvious with the horizontal tube both straight (Fig. 13.3) and slightly curved (Fig. 13.4). While this is not so serious in the larger endotracheal tubes of this type, it can be quite serious in the smallest tubes especially as the amount of protrusion into the lumen varies from tube to tube. When attempting to introduce a catheter into a lumen of 3·0 mm

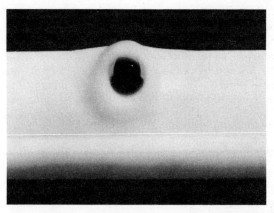

Fig. 13.3. Protrusions in lumen of Jackson Rees tube at level of transverse section.

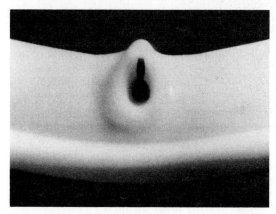

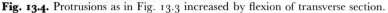

Fig. 13.4. Protrusions as in Fig. 13.3 increased by flexion of transverse section.

one encounters an obstruction at a depth of several centimetres (and not near the surface as in the specially prepared photograph) it can be extremely difficult to aspirate the trachea satisfactorily. An 'Important Notice' is placed in the packet with the tube, pointing out the hazard of allowing the horizontal tube to flex in the direction shown in Fig. 13.4. The Notice recommends that the horizontal tube be fixed in such a manner that it tends to curve in the opposite direction to that shown in Fig. 13.4.

Subglottic oedema and subglottic stenosis

This has been the most serious of all complications and it occurred so consistently in some series that it appeared to be unavoidable. One encouraging factor suggesting it was not inevitable was the low incidence (approximately 5%) in one series. A widely held current view is that the tubes used in the earlier series were, in a few cases, too large.

In paediatric anaesthetic practice one uses the largest tube which will easily pass the larynx and this results in an airtight fit. While this is satisfactory for relatively short periods, it is probably not so for intubation lasting more than 24 hours. To err on the side of safety, Stocks (1970) recommends that the correct size of tube is 0·5 mm internal diameter less than the size which gives an airtight fit. To the less experienced a useful guide is that when positive pressure is applied to the tube to inflate the lungs there should be an audible leak around the tube at laryngeal level. It is this leak which leads to difficulty in using the pneumotachograph to measure pulmonary volumes.

The endotracheal tube, unlike plastic tubes in the urethra or oesophagus, must pass a non-distensible area at the level of the cricoid cartilage. Any pressure on the mucosa at this level must lead to ischaemia, oedema and, ultimately, fibrosis. Treatment of a severe stenosis is extremely difficult and a long-term tracheostomy lasting over a period of years is the unfortunate outcome.

These complications have been dealt with at length because they are, on the whole, preventable and because the consequences of complications occurring are extremely serious and often fatal.

Tracheostomy

Tracheostomy is now used in the management of both upper and lower airway problems. In the past decade, whilst experience has built up with prolonged endotracheal intubation, the management of tracheostomy has improved enormously. Complications such as death during the operative procedure, blockage or dislodgment of the tracheostomy tube, pneumothorax, tracheal stenosis and delayed decannulation are largely preventable (Fearon, 1962; Holinger et al., 1965; Aberdeen, 1965; Glover, 1970a, b).

As in prolonged endotracheal intubation, attention to detail is extremely important because complications, usually preventable, are so serious.

Technique

Anaesthesia

Formerly, tracheostomy in young children was often performed as an emergency under local anaesthesia, sometimes in the ward rather than the operating theatre. There was a high operative mortality from asphyxia, and other operative complications such as pneumothorax were understandably high. Today, in almost all centres, general anaesthesia via an endotracheal tube is employed. This ensures a good airway and a well oxygenated, motionless patient enabling a planned operation to proceed without haste. The abolition of respiratory obstruction results in less tendency for the apex of the pleura to herniate into the wound, thus greatly minimizing the danger of pneumothorax.

If the situation presents as an emergency, then an endotracheal tube should be passed as this enables the operation to take place as an elective procedure.

Surgical aspects

The most likely cause for decannulation difficulties is failure to observe certain well established surgical principles. There are two important points to observe:

1. The first tracheal ring should be left intact as division of it can lead to perichondritis and subglottic stenosis (Watts, 1963).

2. No cartilage should be excised, especially in the infant trachea. If cartilage is excised it does not regenerate and healing is by fibrous tissue with consequent narrowing (Watts, 1963).

These points can be met by making a vertical incision in the mid-line of the trachea through the third and fourth (Holinger et al., 1965), or third, fourth and fifth tracheal rings (Aberdeen, 1968). The tracheostomy tube is then inserted and fixed by means of tapes round the neck. It is important to flex the neck fully when the tapes are being secured as the distance from the tracheostomy to the posterior aspect of the neck is minimal in this position. Failure to flex the neck fully at this stage will result in the tapes being inadequately tightened, with serious danger of dislodgment of the tube on return to the ward. If the tapes are at the correct tension then plastic foam should be placed between them and the back of the neck to avoid trauma to the skin.

Tracheostomy tube

Some years ago the most commonly used tube in infants was the silver cannula with a removable inner tube. The removable inner tube was to enable a blocked tracheostomy tube to be cleared. If humidification is adequate, as described earlier, then blockage of the tube should be extremely rare. There are two disadvantages to these metal tubes:

1. The rigid tube cannot adapt to the trachea and therefore pressure will occur at certain points. Pressure may occur on a tracheal ring, leading to necrosis of cartilage with subsequent collapse of the trachea when decannulation is attempted. Pressure may also occur where the tip of the tube is in contact with the trachea and this may cause ulceration of the tracheal wall anteriorly or laterally, leading sometimes to erosion of an adjacent vessel. If ulceration of the trachea occurs posteriorly a tracheo-oesophageal fistula may develop.

2. The removable inner tube seriously encroaches on the lumen in infant tubes. It is then more difficult to introduce a suction catheter and it is also more difficult to ventilate the lungs because of the high resistance of the narrow lumen.

Most centres now use plastic tracheostomy tubes. The tube designed by Aberdeen (1965) has been very satisfactory (Stool et al., 1968; Talbert and Haller, 1968). It is marketed as the 'Great Ormond Street tracheostomy tube' (Fig. 13.5). Tubes of this type adapt to the individual infant's trachea without causing excessive pressure at any point.

A very important point concerning tracheostomy tubes in infants and

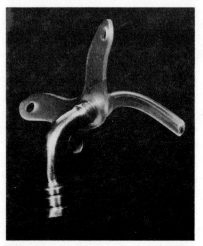

Fig. 13.5. Great Ormond Street tracheostomy tube with connector.

young children is that an inflatable cuff is unnecessary. By putting in the largest tracheostomy tube which will comfortably fit the trachea one has a sufficiently leak-proof fit to be clinically satisfactory and to enable high inflating pressures to be used if required. There is ample evidence now that inflatable cuffs increase the incidence of tracheal trauma (Lunding, 1964; Robertson, 1964; Stiles, 1965).

Management

Many of the important points in management are similar to those for a patient on a ventilator or a patient with an indwelling endotracheal tube; for example, a special nurse is required, good humidification is essential and care in fixing the tube to avoid dislodgment must be ensured.

If the patient shows any respiratory embarrassment after the tracheostomy tube is in place, one must exclude the possibility of a pneumothorax. A pneumothorax may occur preoperatively if respiratory obstruction is present or it may occur at the time the tracheostomy is being performed if the apex of the pleura herniates into the wound.

Changing the tracheostomy tube

With good humidification it is seldom necessary to change the tube frequently. The usual routine is to change it once per week to enable more complete toilet to be carried out to the stoma. It should be changed in the operating theatre in the first three days as it may be extremely difficult to replace it before a track has formed.

Prevention of infection

The danger of infection is greatest in very young infants, especially premature babies. On the rare occasions that premature babies have a tracheostomy the greatest care should be taken to avoid infection; for example, sterile gloves should be worn for tracheal aspiration which must be performed with a sterile catheter. However, in infants even a few weeks old there is much less danger from this source. Indeed, many such infants already carry pathogens such as *Pseudomonas aeruginosa*, or coagulase-positive staphylococci in their nose, throat or rectum. These organisms will almost inevitably be isolated subsequently from tracheal aspirate after a tracheostomy. Nevertheless, these patients usually do not appear clinically infected and it is probably unwise to treat such patients with antibiotics in the absence of clinical signs. One should use a 'no-touch' technique in aspirating the trachea of these older infants.

Decannulation

If tracheostomy has been performed as described and if a plastic tracheostomy tube has been used, then, provided the upper airway was normal before the tracheostomy, one does not anticipate difficulty in decannulation. The commonest cause of decannulation difficulty is a tracheostomy which affects the first ring of the trachea.

Before attempting decannulation one must ensure that the infant is in a satisfactory respiratory condition; namely, that secretions are minimal and that cardiac failure or other cause of respiratory difficulty has been eliminated.

One peculiar feature of young infants is that they often fail to breathe satisfactorily through their normal airway immediately after decannulation. This may be due to an inco-ordination affecting the larynx and developing after tracheostomy; i.e. the glottis tends to close on inspiration. The infant then struggles for air and becomes cyanosed as the stoma closes and a vicious cycle is set up.

A successful method of overcoming this phenomenon is to sedate the infant fairly heavily with morphine (0·2 mg/kg) and remove the tracheostomy tube. Usually the sedated infant continues to sleep, the stoma closes gradually and as it closes more and more air is inspired via the nose. By the time the infant is fully awake, in two to three hours, respiration is well established through the normal passages and the stoma may be almost closed.

One important warning must be given. If, in spite of sedation, an infant shows signs of airway obstruction as the stoma closes, one must consider that there is an organic obstruction until proved otherwise. The safest procedure is to replace the tracheostomy and to do an elective tracheoscopy under general anaesthesia to exclude granulations or a mucosal flap at the site of the stoma.

Summary

Large series of infants have now been managed either by prolonged endotracheal intubation or by tracheostomy in a number of centres. Neither method is easy because simple mistakes with either can so easily be fatal, especially in ill patients.

From the nursing aspect an endotracheal tube seems more difficult to manage and is less pleasant for the patient. The problem of preventing erosion of the ala of the nose becomes more difficult with time. Finally, the serious complication of subglottic stenosis, while probably related to the use of too large a tube as already described, may also be related to duration of intubation. For these reasons the case for intubation becomes weaker the longer the tube is required in a particular patient.

A tracheostomy does, however, involve a small operation and a small scar on the neck. In a few patients granulations may form in the trachea at the level of the stoma and if the procedure has been performed at too high a level there will be decannulation difficulties.

A reasonable conclusion is that in a patient requiring an artificial airway for about two weeks an endotracheal tube should be used provided an audible leak of gas around the tube exists on application of positive pressure (Battersby et al., 1976). If, after this time, it becomes apparent that he is not improving rapidly so that extubation can be done then it is probably advisable to do a tracheostomy at that stage.

Both methods have made considerable contributions to the care of ill patients and each method should be regarded as complementing the other rather than excluding it.

References

Abbott, T. R. (1968). Complications of prolonged nasotracheal intubation in children. *Brit. J. Anaesth.* **40**, 347.

Aberdeen, E. (1965). Mechanical pulmonary ventilation in infants. Tracheostomy and tracheostomy care in infants. *Proc. roy. Soc. Med.* **58**, 900.

Aberdeen, E. (1968). In: *Operative Surgery*. Vol. 2, *Thorax*, 2nd edn. Ed. by W. P. Cleland. London and Boston, Mass., Butterworths.

Allen, L. P., Blake, A. M., Durbin, G. M., Ingram, D., Reynolds, E. O. R. and Wimberley, P. D. (1975). Continuous positive airway pressure and mechanical ventilation by facemask in newborn infants. *Brit. med. J.* **4**, 137.

Allen, T. H. and Steven, I. M. (1965). Prolonged endotracheal intubation in infants and children. *Brit. J. Anaesth.* **37**, 566.

Battersby, E. F., Hatch, D. J. and Towey, R. M. (1977). The effects of prolonged naso-endotracheal intubation in children. *Anaesthesia* **32**, 154.

Bolton, D. P. G. and Cross, K. W. (1974). Further observations on cost of preventing retrolental fibroplasia. *Lancet* **1**, 445.

Brandstater, B. (1962). *Proc. First European Congress of Anaesthesiology, Paper 106*. Excerpta Medica, Vienna.

Chamney, A. R. (1969). Humidification requirements and techniques. Including a review of the performance of equipment in current use. *Anaesthesia* **24**, 602.

Cross, K. W. (1965). *Handbook of Physiology, section 3, Respiration*, Vol. II. Washington, DC, American Physiological Society.

Cross, K. W. (1973). Cost of preventing retrolental fibroplasia? *Lancet* **2**, 954.

Dalhamn, T. (1956). Mucous flow and ciliary activity in trachea of healthy rats, etc. *Acta physiol. scand.* **36**, Suppl. 123.

Fearon, B. (1962). Acute laryngotracheobronchitis in infancy and childhood. *Pediat. Clin. N. Amer.* **9**, 1095.

Galloway, T. C. (1943). Tracheostomy in bulbar poliomyelitis *J. Amer. med. Assoc.* **123**, 1096.

Glover, W. J. (1965). Mechanical ventilation in respiratory insufficiency in infants. *Proc. roy. Soc. Med.* **58**, 902.

Glover, W. J. (1970a). Nasotracheal intubation and tracheostomy in intensive care of infants. *Acta anaesth. scand.* Suppl. **37**, 62.

Glover, W. J. (1970b). Paediatric intensive care. *Progress in Anaesthesiology*, International congress Series, No. 200, p. 451. Excerpta Medica Foundation, Amsterdam.

Gregory, G. A., Kitterman, J. A., Phibbs, R. H., Tooley, W. H. and Hamilton, W. K. (1971). Treatment of the idiopathic respiratory-distress syndrome with continuous positive airway pressure. *New Engl. J. Med.* **284**, 1333.

Guess, W. L. and Stetson, J. B. (1968). Tissue reactions to organotinstabilized polyvinyl chloride (PVC) catheters. *J. Amer. med. Assoc.* **204**, 580.

Hatch, D. J. (1968). Prolonged nasotracheal intubation in infants and children. *Lancet* **1**, 1272.

Hogg, J. C., Williams, J., Richardson, J. B., Macklem, P. T. and Thurlbeck, W. M. (1970). Age as a factor in the distribution of lower-airway conductance and in the pathologic anatomy of obstructive lung disease. *New Engl. J. Med.* **282**, 1283.

Holinger, P. H., Brown, W. T. and Maurizi, D. G. (1965). Tracheostomy in the newborn. *Amer. J. Surg.* **109**, 771.

Jackson Rees, G. and Owen-Thomas, J. B. (1966). A technique of pulmonary ventilation with a nasotracheal tube. *Brit. J. Anaesth.* **38**, 901.

Lunding, M. (1964). The tracheostomy tube and postoperative tracheostomy complications with special reference to severe arterial bleeding caused by erosion of the innominate artery. *Acta anaesth. scand.* **8**, 181.

McDonald, I. H. and Stocks, J. G. (1965). Prolonged nasotracheal intubation. A review of its development in a paediatric hospital. *Brit. J. Anaesth.* **37**, 161.

Modell, J. H., Moya, F., Ruiz, B. C., Showers, A. V. and Newby, E. J. (1968). Blood gas and electrolyte determinations during exposure to ultrasonic nebulized aerosols. *Brit. J. Anaesth.* **40**, 20.

Mushin, W. W., Rendell-Baker, L., Thompson, P. W. and Mapleson, W. W. (1969). *Automatic Ventilation of the Lungs.* Blackwell Scientific Publications, Oxford.

Report of the Committee on Fetus and Newborn of the American Academy of Pediatrics (1971). Oxygen therapy in the newborn infant. *Pediatrics* **47**, 1086.

Robertson, D. S. (1964). Tracheostomy and open heart surgery. *Proc. roy. Soc. Med.* **57**, 855.

Stiles, P. J. (1965). Tracheal lesions after tracheostomy. *Thorax* **20**, 517.

Stocks, J. G. (1970). Paediatric intensive care. *Progress in Anaesthesiology*, International Congress Series, No. 200, p. 517. Excerpta Medica Foundation, Amsterdam.

Stool, S. E., Campbell, J. R. and Johnson, D. G. (1968). Tracheostomy in children: the use of plastic tubes. *J. pediat. Surg.* **3**, 402.

Swensson, S. A. (1962). Management of the Engstrom respirator in early infancy. *Arch. Dis. Childh.* **37**, 156.

Talbert, J. L. and Haller, J. A. (1968). Improved silastic tracheostomy tubes for infants and young children. *J. pediat. Surg.* **3**, 408.

Watts, J. McK. (1963). Tracheostomy in modern practice. *Brit. J. Surg.* **50**, 954.

Wolfsdorf, J., Swift, D. L. and Avery, M. E. (1969). Mist therapy reconsidered; an evaluation of the respiratory deposition of labelled water aerosols produced by jet and ultrasonic nebulizers. *Pediatrics* **43**, 799.

Chapter 14

Measurements during Artificial Ventilation and their Significance

Examination

With the development of sophisticated, expensive monitoring apparatus it has become increasingly apparent that the simplest and most satisfactory comprehensive monitoring of the patient is the result of intelligent observation by experienced personnel.

Observation of the patient will provide information about his state of consciousness, and from the colour of his skin we can make an estimate of the adequacy of the vascular perfusion of the skin and the amount of reduced haemoglobin in his capillary bed. A cyanosed patient is nearly always a patient in whom hypoxia is present, or in whom cardiac output is insufficient to meet the metabolic demands of the tissues.

The patient's demeanour may give an indication of the state of cerebral oxygenation. Any patient who exhibits restlessness should be suspected of suffering from cerebral hypoxia, whether this be the result of insufficient oxygen in his arterial blood or insufficient circulation to his brain. Conversely, it would be most unusual for a patient with gross disturbance of his physiology to be cerebrating normally.

By observing the movement of the chest one can make an assessment of the adequacy of ventilation and one can detect inequality between the movement of the right and left side of the chest, indicative of uneven pulmonary ventilation or intubation of the right main bronchus.

Distension of the veins may indicate cardiac failure or overhydration, and the presence or absence of oedema may help to determine whether this diagnosis is to be substantiated.

Useful information can be obtained by listening to the patient's breathing. Expiratory wheezing or inspiratory stridor can warn the attendant staff of developing bronchospasm or an obstructed airway. One can frequently detect coarse râles associated with sputum in the larger bronchi or in the tracheostomy tube. Detection of finer râles, indicating sputum present in the smaller bronchi and alveoli, requires auscultation of the chest with a stethoscope. Listening may also allow one to detect the leakage of gas past a poorly fitting tracheostomy tube or inadequately inflated cuff, which may result in insufficient alveolar ventilation. To the experienced observer a change in the noise of the ventilator may indicate a change in the ventilatory pattern.

There is no single measurement that can provide a definitive description of any physiological disturbances. It is only by making a series of observations on multiple parameters that useful information can be achieved. Generally it is the trend of change revealed by sequential measurements that indicates the patient's response to therapy; hence the necessity of charting all observations against a time scale. This emphasizes the importance of keeping adequate intensive care unit charts and displaying information on a 24-hour chart.

Measurements of ventilation

Ultimately the adequacy of ventilation will depend upon the efficient way in which oxygen is added to the blood and carbon dioxide is removed. There is, therefore, no true substitute for arterial blood-gas estimates although measurements performed on alveolar gas samples and venous blood will provide useful information. However, these estimates are not usually made continuously but intermittently, and between the time that they are made one must be able to follow the path of the ventilation constantly. For this reason it is necessary to record the rate of ventilation together with the volume that is exhaled from the patient at each breath. There are many dry gas meters available to measure the exhaled volume, but the Wright respirometer (see Fig. 11.1), is sufficiently accurate for clinical use although great care is required to ensure that it does not become waterlogged by condensation of exhaled moisture. The product of pump rate per minute and exhaled tidal volume will give the patient's minute volume. Provided that there is not a great change in the state of the patient's pulmonary condition then a constant minute volume will reflect constant alveolar ventilation and the maintenance of a safe degree of oxygenation and removal of carbon dioxide. In the long-term management of patients on ventilators, especially those with normal pulmonary function, it often suffices to follow the ventilatory parameters, only performing alveolar or blood-gas analysis if there is a change in their physical status.

It is important to appreciate the relationship between tidal volume and dead space. A certain proportion of each breath will not take part in ventilating those areas of the lung where gaseous exchange takes place; this constitutes the dead space ventilation. Some of this dead space may be due to gases being breathed in and out of endotracheal tubes, catheter mounts or facemasks—this constitutes anatomical or apparatus dead space; the rest is due to inspired gas ventilating parts of the lungs that are poorly perfused and hence only part of this gas volume takes part in gaseous exchange. The higher the proportion of the tidal volume (Vt) that ventilates dead space (VD), the greater the VD/Vt ratio, and thus less effective will be the ventilation at a given minute volume. An increasing VD/Vt as indicated by an increase in the Pa_{CO_2} at a constant ventilatory minute volume, using the same apparatus, suggests that an increasing proportion of the lung is being ventilated without being adequately perfused. This occurs if the inflating pressure is increased due to a fall in pulmonary compliance, if positive end-expiratory pressure (PEEP) is introduced, if the patient's cardiac output decreases or he becomes hypovolaemic and if there is a pulmonary embolus.

Changes in Pa_{O_2} are similarly of significance in the presence of a constant ventilatory minute volume. A fall in Pa_{O_2} without a concomitant change in Pa_{CO_2} suggests that, although alveolor ventilation remains constant, less blood is being oxygenated; this is usually due to an increasing proportion of the pulmonary blood flow being shunted past alveoli that are not being adequately ventilated—an increase in 'shunt blood'. This can be confirmed by estimating the alveolar–arterial oxygen gradient $(PA–a_{O_2})$. In the clinical situation estimate of alveolar oxygen tension can be made using the simplified alveolar air equation. This requires knowing the alveolar Pco_2 and the inspired oxygen tension.

$$PA_{O_2} = PI_{O_2} \frac{Pa_{CO_2}}{R \cdot Q}$$

For room air and normal alveolar ventilation assuming a respiratory quotient of 0·8:

$$PA_{O_2} = 150 \text{ mm Hg} \frac{40 \text{ mm Hg}}{0·8}$$
$$= 100 \text{ mm Hg} *$$

If the blood-gas estimates show a falling Pa_{O_2} in the presence of a relatively normal Pa_{CO_2} then, provided the inspired oxygen concentration has not been changed, it is probable that the patient is shunting a greater proportion of his cardiac output through areas of pulmonary collapse, atelectasis or poorly ventilated alveoli. Examination of the chest and a chest x-ray may reveal the cause; for example, lobar collapse, pneumonic consolidation, intubation of a main bronchus by the tracheostomy or endotracheal tube a developing pulmonary oedema. Frequently, however, there is a tendency for patients receiving artificial ventilation to demonstrate a progressive increase in the alveolar–arterial oxygen difference. This can often be limited or reversed by the use of PEEP, which prevents the alveoli closing down below their critical closing volume during exhalation and so maintains good ventilation of the lung.

This critical closing volume tends to be larger in older patients, requiring a higher critical closing pressure to prevent alveoli from closing. The tendency to this progressive increase in the amount of blood shunted past the underventilated alveoli is increased by cigarette smoking.

It is useful to follow the peak pressure reached during inspiration, and ventilators should incorporate a manometer dial to allow this measurement to be recorded. Changes in the pressure required to achieve a set tidal volume will indicate changes in compliance of the system. This may draw one's attention to a blockage of the delivery tubing and an increase in secretion of sputum, small airways obstruction or a lesser degree of relaxation of the chest wall. This should always be a warning sign that some change has taken place that might require immediate attention. It is often the earliest indication that an overlong tracheostomy tube has entered the

* Using SI units:
$$PA_{O_2} = 20 \text{ kPa} - \frac{5·3 \text{ kPa}}{0·8} = 13·3 \text{ kPa}$$

right main bronchus, obstructing gas flow into the left lung, or that a plug of sputum has lodged in the tracheostomy tube. The combination of information regarding changes in inflation pressure, minute volume and blood gases will help one differentiate between the various causes of a change in dead space.

Temperature

Because of the vulnerability of the tracheostomized patient to infection, it is essential that attention is paid to any change in the patient's temperature. The temperature should be recorded six-hourly. Any increase in the patient's temperature should draw attention to the possibility of pulmonary infection although one must bear in mind other possible sites of infection, and in the case of brain injury it may represent mid-brain damage.

Blood pressure, pulse and central venous pressure

The blood pressure and pulse rate should be recorded every 15–30 minutes in patients on ventilators.

A change in these parameters may indicate an alteration in cardiac output or in peripheral resistance. Changes in cardiac output may be secondary to alterations in intrathoracic pressure or failure of the venous return. A change in peripheral resistance might be a result of increased absorption of a central depressant drug in a patient who has narcotic poisoning or a worsening of a patient's intracranial disease. It can also be caused by progressive spinal disease. The usefulness of central venous pressure measurements using a catheter inserted into the superior or inferior vena cava is now well established. The catheter may be inserted direct into the internal jugular vein in the neck by a puncture performed between the sternal and clavicular heads of the sternomastoid muscle, via the subclavian vein which is best entered by a puncture just below the clavicle or through the basilic or cephalic veins. If a peripheral vein is used, an x-ray should confirm the central position of the catheter tip. A CVP catheter line not only serves as a route for the administration of drugs for obtaining venous blood samples, but it also gives a valuable indication of the relationship between venous return and cardiac output. The zero point of these measurements is taken as the level of the manubrium sternum. The venous pressure of the patient on the ventilator should be kept above that of the patient breathing spontaneously so as to allow for the increased intrathoracic pressure. Venous pressures below 5–10 cm H_2O (0·5–1 kPa) probably represent inadequate venous return. In order to assess whether a low cardiac output state is due to failure of venous return or to myocardial depression, a short rapid infusion of 200 ml of fluid may be administered. If the venous pressure rises without an increase in cardiac output and blood pressure, then usually the failure is central in origin. If, however, the cardiac output improves, then there is a positive indication for further transfusion. Like other measurements, it is a change in the recorded values that is of importance in directing attention to changes in the patient's circulatory volume and cardiac function.

Fluid balance

The importance of maintaining a normal fluid balance in patients on ventilators has only recently been realized, especially as the high efficiency of some of the ultrasonic nebulizers can introduce enormous amounts of water into patients without it being recognized on the fluid balance chart. Patients at special risk should therefore be weighed daily. An increase in a patient's weight in spite of good urinary output may indicate water retention due to inhaled water; this is especially likely to be the cause if there is an associated fall in pulmonary compliance. This condition should be treated with diuretics. Urinary output should be monitored. The blood urea, the specific gravity of the urine and, in the immediate postoperative period, the sodium and potassium content of the urine, may be helpful in following the function of the kidneys during the time the patient is on positive pressure ventilation. This information is of help in directing replacement therapy.

Haemoglobin

The oxygen content of the blood will depend not only upon the alveolar ventilation and the partial pressure of oxygen in the alveoli but also upon the capacity of blood to carry oxygen. The oxygen content of the arterial blood (in ml) will be the product of $1.34 \times O_2$ saturation $\times$ Hb content (g). The occurrence of any significant anaemia can be deleterious to these patients. Because these patients are often being fed by intravenous means for long periods, it is important to follow their haematocrit and to correct any anaemia that may occur. Similarly, plasma proteins may be reduced as a result of insufficient protein intake in the diet provided or excessive neoglucogenesis in response to inadequate calorie intake.

Serum electrolytes

Patients on ventilators should have their serum electrolytes estimated every day so that electrolyte intake for the subsequent 24 hours can be correctly assessed. This regimen can be modified for patients stabilized on long-term artificial ventilation, especially if they are eating a normal diet.

Chest x-rays

A patient should have an erect chest x-ray after a tracheostomy has been performed. This should check the position of the tube to determine whether it has entered one bronchus and whether a pneumothorax has been produced.

It is advisable for patients on ventilators to have daily chest x-rays. However, if this becomes impracticable or dangerous, as in long-term artificial ventilation, then chest x-rays less frequently must suffice. Any patient in whom a tracheostomy has recently been performed should have a chest x-ray to ensure that both lungs are expanded.

ECG and pulse

The continuous display of an ECG is a reassuring sign that cardiac activity continues; however, by itself it does not denote the adequacy of that activity. It must be appreciated that a normal single-lead ECG does not mean that there have not been changes in cardiac function or in cardiac output. Similarly, the ECG may be abnormal yet the cardiac output may be sufficient. Changes in ECG pattern rhythm and rate do, however, indicate an altered physiological status which should alert the attendant. The ECG pattern may alter because of hypoxia, poor coronary artery perfusion, electrolyte change or acid–base changes. The rate may increase to compensate for a decrease in stroke volume of the heart or it may indicate a wearing off of the central effect of sedative drugs. Changes in the ECG may be the first sign of ventricular irritability leading to extrasystoles, ventricular fibrillation and cardiac arrest. Generally, ventricular arrythmias are of more serious import than sinus or atrial changes.

The pulse, monitored at the wrist or ear, gives an indication of tissue blood flow; it is difficult to envisage a situation in which a good pulse was monitored in the presence of an inadequate cardiac output.

The duration of the time interval between the QRS complex of the ECG (signalling ventricular activity) and the arrival of the pulse at the wrist will vary with the force of ventricular contraction and the velocity of the pulse wave in that patient. As the latter is fairly constant in clinical circumstances, changes in the time interval between the QRS complex of the ECG and the arrival of the pulse at the wrist gives a reasonable indirect measurement of myocardial performance. Prolongation of this interval (the systolic time interval) indicates a failing myocardium.

Blood gases

It is inadvisable to undertake the treatment of patients by artificial ventilation unless facilities for blood-gas analysis are available. Patients on ventilators should have estimates of their arterial P_{CO_2}, P_{O_2}, pH and serum bicarbonate made repeatedly.

This can be achieved with either a pH meter and a CO_2 and O_2 electrode or by means of an Astrup apparatus. The Astrup apparatus is based on a pH meter. The pH of the blood sample is determined at the same P_{CO_2} as that at which it was withdrawn. The blood sample is then equilibrated with a gas mixture containing a known high P_{CO_2} and the pH again determined. The process is repeated by equilibrating the sample with CO_2 at a known low P_{CO_2} before again determining the pH. The two pH determinations at known P_{CO_2} levels are then plotted on semi-log paper and the points joined. By interpolating the original pH reading on this line it is possible to read off the P_{CO_2} of the original sample, and by relating the line to a family of lines (isopleths) the base deficit can be determined (Fig. 14.1).

Any alteration in the setting of the ventilatory parameters should be followed within half an hour by an estimate of the blood gases to observe the magnitude of any change that might occur in the patient's arterial blood. It is only by following the patient's arterial oxygen and the Pco_2 that

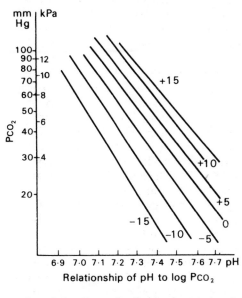

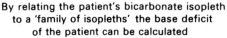

Relationship of pH to log Pco_2

By relating the patient's bicarbonate isopleth
to a 'family of isopleths' the base deficit
of the patient can be calculated

Fig. 14.1. Astrup plot of log Pco_2 against pH. This produced a bicarbonate 'isopleth'.

the efficacy of the ventilation can be assessed, although a useful index of the adequacy of the alveolar ventilation can be achieved by estimating the Pa_{CO_2} (alveolar CO_2). During the period when the patient is being weaned from the ventilator it is necessary to observe repeatedly the response of the patient's blood gases. Any tendency of the Pco_2 to rise above 60 mm Hg (8 kPa) should be an indication for the patient to be returned to artificial ventilation.

The pH of the patient on artificial ventilation should be kept as near to 7·4 as possible. It is important to correct any gross base (bicarbonate) deficit that may be revealed by this estimation. The ratio of the Pco_2 to the bicarbonate content determines the hydrogen ion concentration (pH) of the tissue fluids. A base deficit greater than 3 mmol/l, at normal body temperature, should be corrected. It is imperative that the hydrogen ion concentration of the patient is kept within narrow limits if bodily processes are to proceed normally. Gross acidaemia or alkalaemia produces depression of the central nervous system, the circulation, respiration, metabolism and renal excretion. A low plasma bicarbonate is the result of either:

1. an excess production of fixed (metabolic) acids, or
2. an excessive loss of base from the body.

An excess production of fixed acids, particularly lactic acid, results from anaerobic conditions and the conversion of pyruvic to lactic acid as a means of oxidizing the metabolic enzyme $NADH_2$. Ultimately the lactic acid is metabolized to CO_2 and H_2O when oxygen is once more available. Anaerobic metabolism occurs wherever the oxygen demands of the tissue outstrip the available oxygen. During circulatory arrest, following cardiac arrest, anaerobic metabolism produces metabolic acidaemia that is apparent on re-establishing the circulation. During haemorrhagic shock, when hypotension and vasoconstriction combine to produce inadequate tissue perfusion, lactacidaemia is produced. It is also found after anoxic and hypoxic episodes, hypotension, following obstruction to the circulation to large muscle masses, during shivering and cardiac pulmonary bypass. Ketone acids are produced by the incomplete metabolism of fats, due to the non-availability of carbohydrate intermediate metabolites. It occurs in diabetic ketonaemia and it also produces a metabolic acidosis.

An excessive loss of base results from the unreplaced loss of the secretions of the upper intestinal tract and pancreatic juices. Chronic intestinal obstruction is often associated with metabolic acidosis. Renal loss of base also occurs, although the normal secretion of the kidney is acid. It is nearly always found following ureteric transplantation.

Base deficit may be corrected by giving NaCl, provided the patient is able to excrete the Cl^- radical and conserve the base. This process takes time, and needs a fluid load and good renal function. Ringer lactate solution can be used to correct a base deficit, but this will depend upon the metabolism of the lactate by the liver and the conservation of the base. Once again, this process takes time. The best method of rapidly correcting a base deficit of sufficient magnitude to produce symptoms is by giving sodium bicarbonate 8·4% solution. This solution contains 0·5 mmol/l of bicarbonate. As the base is given as its sodium salt, it will be primarily distributed in the patients extracellular water—a volume that corresponds to 25% of his body weight in kg. However, if the cause of the base deficit was an excessive production of fixed acids, it is likely that the base deficit will be both intracellular and extracellular. In these circumstances 25% of body weight times the base deficit will result in inadequate replacement and one must be prepared to give about double this amount of bicarbonate during the replacement period. In this circumstance it is well to give the initial infusion of bicarbonate of 25% of body weight times the base deficit fairly rapidly (10 min to 1 hour) and to continue to give bicarbonate slowly for the next 12 hours whilst equilibration is taking place across the cell membrane. It is advisable always to follow massive bicarbonate therapy by repeated blood-gas, pH and bicarbonate estimates. Frequently a rise in Pco_2 follows the administration of bicarbonate, necessitating increased ventilation.

If a patient is unconscious then great care is needed and it is advisable to perform acid–base measurements frequently; at a minimum these should be carried out every day. However, with patients on long-term artificial ventilation in whom these parameters have become stabilized it may suffice with pH, bicarbonate and P$_{CO_2}$ estimates being made less frequently. Only when the patient has full consciousness and is able to inform his attendants that his ventilation feels adequate and it can be observed that he does not exhibit the effects of hypoxia or hypercarbia, can the blood gases be safely ignored for longer periods.

Alveolar CO$_2$

In situations where blood-gas analysis is not available or to obviate the necessity for repeated arterial sampling, it is possible to obtain useful information about the adequacy of alveolar ventilation by measuring the alveolar P$_{CO_2}$ (P$_{A_{CO_2}}$). A sample of this gas may be obtained by filling a 500 ml anaesthetic bag (child's size) with oxygen, connecting it to the tracheostomy by a catheter mount and Nosworthy connection, and ventilating the patient with the contents of the bag for 20 seconds. The bag is then clamped off at the end of expiration. Five minutes later the process is repeated. At the end of this time the contents of the bag will have equilibrated with that in the patient's alveoli. Analysis of the gas for CO$_2$ will give a measure of alveolar CO$_2$. This analysis can be carried out simply at the bedside with a Campbell-modified Haldane apparatus or an infrared CO$_2$ analyser.

In addition to these specific measurements which may be made on all patients on ventilators, certain additional information may be required according to the disease process that necessitated the patient's admission to the intensive care unit and his treatment by artificial ventilation. Thus if the patient has a condition associated with instability of cardiac rhythm, in addition to monitoring the ECG and pulse it may be desirable to use an electronic cardiorater and cardiac alarm system. In patients with severe head injuries, it may be desirable to closely monitor signs of changes in levels of consciousness, the size and responsiveness of the pupils, the patient's reflexes and his responsiveness to stimuli. Similarly, in postoperative patients other parameters such as urine output, fluid intake, haemoglobin, plasma proteins and electrolytes may become important. It is important that patients who are being treated for ventilatory insufficiency on artificial ventilation should at the same time receive complete supportive therapy, as it is only too easy for the attendant to become so engrossed by his interest in the patient's ventilation that he fails to treat the patient as a whole.

In all measurements it is easy to forget that every investigation disturbs the patient, some carry a morbidity and a few have caused the patient's death. Useless and inappropriate measurements should not be made because of any routine without considering the likely value of the information derived. It is axiomatic that multiple measurements cannot be used as a substitute for good clinical care—no patient has been restored to health as a result of any measurement; it is the sensible utilization of the information derived from these measurements that benefits the patient.

Chapter 15

Infection—Epidemiology, Prevention and Treatment

Tracheostomy and artificial ventilation are inevitably an integral part of intensive care and it is in the setting of the intensive care unit that we must examine the problems of infection. Recent years have seen an exponential proliferation of sophisticated equipment and treatments with a consequential increase in the problems of preventing and treating infection. Patients requiring intensive care nowadays are more likely to have undergone major surgery resulting in alterations to normal anatomy and physiology; more likely to have been given broad spectrum antibiotics resulting in alterations to normal body flora; and more likely to have received steroids or cytotoxics resulting in alterations to normal host defence mechanisms. For all these reasons patients in the intensive care unit are unusually susceptible to infection, and the accumulation of a number of such 'compromised hosts' in a small specialized area can produce a very high and unacceptable level of infection. For these patients who are already dangerously ill, but who may have a reasonable chance of recovery, an otherwise minor infection may be the final insult.

In order to be better able to understand the microbiological problems of intensive care it is first necessary to be familiar with the ways in which microbes spread and cause disease and the reasons why the patient in the ICU is more susceptible to infection. Armed with this knowledge one can then take rational steps to prevent and treat infection.

Factors influencing the occurrence of infection

Micro-organisms are ubiquitous. They may be free living in soil or water and generally harmless to man. They may be **commensal** micro-organisms living in large numbers harmlessly in or on the body and are non-pathogenic provided they do not stray from the site in which they constitute part of the normal body flora.

Examples of commensal bacteria are *Staphylococcus epidermidis* and diphtheroids on skin, *Streptococcus viridans* in the oral cavity, and the coliform group of organisms, such as *Escherichia coli*, and the anaerobic organisms, such as Bacteroides, in the alimentary tract. These **potential pathogens**, normally harmless and in some cases beneficial to the host, can cause infection if they colonize a normally sterile body site as a result of some invasive procedure or diminished host defences. Examples of this include postcatheterization urinary tract infection caused by intestinal *E. coli*, drip-site infection by *Staph. epidermidis* and tracheostomy or pulmonary infection by *E. coli*, Klebsiella or *Pseudomonas aeruginosa*.

Some organisms, such as *P. aeruginosa*, which are normally non-pathogenic and rarely cause disease in the normal individual, are termed **opportunistic pathogens**. They cause trouble only where host defences are weakened either medically or surgically. Opportunistic infections are often severe and difficult to treat unless the underlying abnormality can be corrected.

Very few bacteria encountered in the ICU are pathogens *per se*. Only rarely are organisms such as *Bacillus anthracis*, the causative organism of anthrax, or *Clostridium tetani* (which causes tetanus) found. If they are, one can safely assume that they were not hospital-acquired.

Clinical determinants of hospital-acquired infection

Age

Patients who are very young or very old are more liable to infection. Although age in itself is important, the non-infectious illnesses peculiar to patients at the extremes of age are probably even more important.

Obesity

Patients who are extremely obese are more prone to postoperative infection than others.

Foreign bodies

Catheters, cannulae, sutures and prostheses for insertion into various orifices, organs and tissues, for diagnostic or therapeutic purposes, can carry potential pathogens deep into the host by breaching natural barriers, and infection is the result.

Metabolic factors

Diabetes mellitus is associated with increased susceptibility to infection, possibly due in part to the complications of acidosis, renal dysfunction and cardiovascular insufficiency. Other hormonal disturbances, such as hyper-parathyroidism, may also be associated with a higher incidence of infection.

Steroid therapy

This is frequently associated with increased susceptibility to infection and with the reactivation of latent infection such as tuberculosis. Pyogenic, viral and fungal infections are commoner in patients receiving steroids.

Haematological factors

Patients with leukaemia and lymphoma, characterized by granulocy-topenia or immunological deficiency, are extremely susceptible to infection.

Treatment of the underlying disease also increases the risk and severity of infection.

Immunological factors

Immunosuppression or any deficiency in cellular or humoral immunity increases the risk of infection. Deficiencies of phagocytic cells or lymphocytes, immunoglobulins, complement or other factors, such as lysozyme, all decrease resistance to infection.

Nutritional state

The malnourished or cachectic patient is at greater risk of infection.

Cardiovascular factors

Heart failure, hypotension, shock and ischaemia are important determinants of postoperative infection. Poor tissue perfusion is probably responsible for the greater pathogenicity of otherwise commensal bacteria.

Infective endocarditis following surgery or instrumentation in patients who have congenital or acquired heart disease is an example of the interaction of other factors which belong to this group.

Respiratory factors

Chronic bronchitis, emphysema, bronchiectasis, viral respiratory infections such as influenza, and other destructive, degenerative or suppurative conditions predispose to hospital-acquired pulmonary infection.

Tracheostomy, endotracheal intubation and artificial ventilation bypass nasopharyngeal defences and often result in infection.

Neurological factors

Paralysed patients commonly develop infected pressure sores, and urinary tract infection follows catheterization. Unconscious patients are particularly prone to pneumonia.

Antibiotic factors

The use of broad spectrum antibiotics prophylactically or therapeutically alters body flora and allows superinfection by opportunistic pathogens such as *P. aeruginosa* or Klebsiella.

Miscellaneous factors

The longer the preoperative hospitalization period, the greater is the chance of colonization by hospital organisms and the greater is the chance of subsequent infection. Longer and more complex operations adversely affect postoperative sepsis rates.

'Chance occurrences'

A dose of the potential pathogen sufficient to cause infection must come into contact with an appropriate site in a host who for one reason or another is susceptible to that infection.

Transmission of infection

The origin of any infection may be **endogenous** or **exogenous**. In other words, the offending pathogen may originate from the patient's own bacterial flora or may clearly have come from another, outside source. However, following admission to hospital, patients frequently become colonized by hospital strains of *Staph. aureus*, *E. coli*, Klebsiella and *P. aeruginosa* which may subsequently cause infection. These apparently endogenous infections are in reality exogenous, the patient's alimentary tract, nose or skin being the final pathway leading to infection.

Bacteria are transmitted (and acquired) by one of the following routes:

1. Airborne dissemination.
2. Direct personal contact.
3. Via **fomites**: ingested food, drink, medicaments;
   contaminated solutions and creams;
   instruments and equipment.

The importance of the **airborne route** in the dissemination of micro-organisms which colonize or infect is now well known. This route is particularly important for bacteria which are resistant to drying such as staphylococci, streptococci and tubercle bacilli and for viruses.

Microbes are incapable of becoming airborne and spreading by themselves. They require a carrier of a suitable size that can be swept up on currents of air and remain airborne for a sufficient time to allow contact with potential hosts. Examples of such carriers are particles of dust, desquamated skin scales and minute droplets of secretions such as sputum.

Classically, *Staph. aureus* is shed by carriers on skin scales, with a median diameter of about 13 μm. These bacteria-carrying particles are capable of remaining airborne for long periods and settle out only slowly. They may be trapped during inhalation, resulting in nasal acquisition, or they may settle on bedding or horizontal surfaces in the hospital environment to be acquired by contact.

Mycobacterium tuberculosis is dispersed by small droplet nuclei of sputum, each containing one tubercle bacillus, and respiratory viruses are similarly spread. These minute particles of dried secretions coat and protect the organisms they carry, and when they are inhaled by a susceptible host, infection results. Thus the adage that 'coughs and sneezes spread diseases' is more than an old wives' tale.

Transmission by **direct contact** is also well documented. Both gram-positive cocci and gram-negative bacilli (e.g. coliform organisms) may be spread in this way. The hands of hospital staff, such as nurses, can be contaminated with *Staph. aureus* or *P. aeruginosa* from patients who have been touched and the organisms transmitted to others. Nurses' uniforms and white coats rapidly become contaminated with *Staph. aureus* and other organisms when working with patients and they soon carry a representative sample of the microflora on the ward. This leads to the spread of these organisms from patient to patient.

Fomites (contaminated inanimate objects capable of transmitting infection) are responsible for many outbreaks of hospital infection traceable to a common source. Food and drink, contaminated in the hospital kitchen, and contaminated medicines can produce colonization by *P. aeruginosa* and other bacteria and this may subsequently lead to infection. Other contaminated medicaments such as local anaesthetic or lubricating jellies for tracheal intubation, creams, irrigation fluids and even fluids for intravenous administration can cause colonization, infection or even death. A classic example of a common-source outbreak of hospital infection is that of post-operative *P. aeruginosa* meningitis in neurosurgery caused by contaminated shaving equipment used to prepare the patients. Other equipment, including ventilators, humidifiers, nebulizers and neonatal incubators have been implicated in many outbreaks of hospital infection.

Environmental sources of infection are probably less important than the others. Pseudomonas can be isolated with little difficulty from sink traps and ventilators. However, it is only rarely found in these sites *before* it is found in the patient and so it is probable that these organisms usually pass from patient to environment and only rarely in the reverse direction.

Organisms causing infection

Of the countless bacterial species, only five or six are responsible for the vast majority of hospital infections. It is well known that the spectrum of infection varies from hospital to hospital and from time to time, but these are really minor variations in the relative frequencies of the major pathogens. More than two-thirds of all hospital infections are caused by:

> *Staphylococcus aureus*
> *Escherichia coli*
> Klebsiella
> *Pseudomonas aeruginosa*
> Proteus
> Candida

Of more importance than the identity of these pathogens are their patterns of susceptibility to antibiotics. Hospital-acquired strains of the first five are commonly resistant to a number of antibiotics and some strains may even be resistant to all the commonly available antibacterial agents. As a general rule, selective pressures in the hospital environment determine the nature and antibiotic sensitivity (or resistance) patterns of the major pathogens. If a particular antibiotic is used widely and indiscriminately, and perhaps wrongly, in a particular environment such as the ICU, the pressures will be such that the majority of infections occurring in that unit will be caused by bacteria resistant to the misused antibiotic. A number of such outbreaks have been documented and the result in each, apart from the disastrous consequences to the patients, has been that the unit has had to be closed and restrictions placed on the use of antibiotics.

Candida (yeast) infections rarely occur *ab initio*. They usually occur as superinfections following prolonged broad spectrum antibiotic therapy. On withdrawal of the antibiotics they often clear spontaneously and specific antifungal therapy may not be required.

Bacteroides and other anaerobic bacteria are infrequent pathogens in intensive care.

Control of infection

Because the factors leading to infection are numerous and complex, adequate control of infection can be achieved only by strict adherence to agreed policies covering disinfection and sterilization, antibiotic usage, invasive procedures and nursing procedures, and by the judicious use of common sense. Of vital importance is the education of **all** staff working in intensive care and the maintenance of good communications between them. Only if all the staff work together as a team can the ICU function efficiently, and only if the ICU is functioning efficiently can infection be effectively prevented. It should be remembered that no member of the team, and no visitor to the unit, is too senior or too important to be allowed not to follow the agreed policies.

General policy

Staff working in the ICU for long periods should wear clean, comfortable clothing (such as theatre dress) which is changed at least daily. All other persons entering the unit should remove their outer clothing and put on a gown or apron. Plastic disposable aprons are ideal as they are cheaper than cotton gowns in the long run and are also impervious. Aprons which become contaminated (with blood or pus, for example) must be changed immediately. To enter a cubicle or room housing a patient in protective isolation who is particularly susceptible to infection, the full aseptic ritual, as performed in the operating theatre, should be observed. To enter a containment isolation cubicle (barrier nursing) no special precautions are required. If the infected patient or his bedding is touched, however, or infected material handled, the apron should be discarded into an incineration bag and the hands washed (in that order) before leaving the cubicle. A fresh apron is then put on.

Of major importance in preventing infection is a general restriction of entry to the patient areas. Only personnel essential for a patient's immediate treatment should be allowed entry and large ward rounds must be prohibited. Case discussions can take place in one of the ancillary rooms.

Isolation policy

Protective isolation (reverse barrier nursing)

This is used for patients who are unusually susceptible to infection, such as those on immunosuppressive drugs and cytotoxic agents and those with a low neutrophil count (< 1 000/μl).

Containment isolation (barrier nursing)

This is used for patients with frank infection or who are colonized with a known epidemic strain of a pathogen.

Sterilization

Sterilization is the complete destruction of all types of micro-organisms and is usually achieved by the use of heat or ionizing radiation or ethylene oxide gas. Apart from the last of these, chemical agents cannot be relied upon to sterilize in a short exposure time and physical methods should be used in hospital. These are summarized in Table 15.1.

TABLE 15.1.   STERILIZATION METHODS

Method	Conditions (temperature/time)	Applications
Steam (moist heat)		
Instrument autoclave	134° C/3 min	Unwrapped instruments, bowls and rubber
High vacuum autoclave	134° C/3 min	Dressings, wrapped instruments, rubber
High vacuum autoclave (+ formalin)	70–80° C/15 min (70–80° C/1–3 h)	Pasteurization of heat-sensitive materials: plastics, endoscopes, rubber, specula
Hot water		
Pasteurizer	70–80° C/10 min	Endoscopes, specula, etc.
Dry heat		
Hot air oven	160–180° C/5–60 min	Glass and metal instruments
Incinerator	—	Disposal of infected dressings, linen etc.
Irradiation		
Gamma	2·5 M rads	Heat-sensitive materials, especially plastic disposables
Ethylene oxide	Carefully controlled	Heat-sensitive materials: plastics, endoscopes, electrical equipment

Heat, whether dry or moist, is the most efficient and cheapest method of sterilization and should be used wherever possible. There is an inverse relationship between the temperature used and the time required for sterilization, high temperatures necessitating shorter exposure times. Moist heat kills micro-organisms by coagulation of microbial protein while dry heat causes its oxidative destruction.

Pasteurization (moist heat at 70°–80°C for 10–20 min) kills vegetative organisms (most bacterial pathogens) but it cannot be relied upon to kill spores and viruses. It is thus a method of disinfection rather than sterilization. The addition of formaldehyde to steam at low temperature and pressures in a special autoclave increases the efficiency of the process, and materials treated in this way (e.g. cystoscopes) may be regarded as sterile.

Disinfection

Only physical methods of sterilization, already outlined, can be relied on to kill all microbes. Few liquid disinfectants (if any) kill spores within a reasonable time or viruses with certainty. Their efficiency is reduced by the presence of organic materials, rubber and plastic. Disinfectants should be used **only** where sterilization is impossible, where disposable items are unavailable and where simple cleaning alone will not suffice.

Disinfection may often be accomplished by thorough cleaning, and the best, cheapest and safest method is a combination of cleaning and pasteurization (*v.s.*). Where chemical disinfection cannot be avoided, preparations should be chosen with care as a number of factors affect their performance.

1. *Antibacterial spectrum*. This should be as wide as possible. Some agents (e.g. chloroxylenol (Dettol)) show little activity against gram-negative organisms.

2. *Bacteriostasis*. Organisms are not killed but growth is inhibited. Bactericidal activity is desired.

3. *Temperature*. The higher the temperature, the more effective the disinfection. Dilute with warm water for greater efficiency.

4. *Concentration*. The optimum concentration depends on the degree of contamination and inactivation. It should always be measured and not guessed. Untrained domestic staff cannot be expected to do this without supervision.

5. *Time*. At least 30 minutes is usually necessary.

6. *Inactivation*. The activity of chemical disinfectants is reduced by hard water, organic material (blood, pus, faeces, food), soaps and detergents, cork stoppers and screw-cap liners, and mop-head and mattress-cover materials.

7. *Stability*. Avoid preparing dilutions a long time before use, prolonged keeping in use, and topping up of dilutions and refilling used containers without washing and disinfecting by heat.

Various types of chemical disinfectants are available. The major groups and their properties are summarized below.

1. Phenolics

(*a*) *Black fluids* (e.g. Jeyes' fluid)
(*b*) *White fluids* (e.g. Izal)
(*c*) *Clear soluble fluids* (e.g. Hycolin, Stericol, Sudol, Clearsol)

Wide range of antibacterial activity. Some spores killed. Not much inactivated by organic matter but possibly by plastics. Absorbed by rubber—do not use for facemasks.

(*d*) *Chloroxylenols* (e.g. Dettol)

Effective against gram-positives. Little action against gram-negatives. Not cheap. Greatly inactivated by organic matter.

(*e*) *Hexachlorophane*

Effective against gram-positives. Not cheap. Incorporated in soap and creams. Cumulative effect.

2. Alcohols

Wide range of antibacterial activity. Rapid action. Used alone at 60–90% or with others (chlorhexidine, iodine). Poor penetration of organic matter. Useful for skin or clean surfaces and as aerosol for ventilators. Not cheap.

3. Halogens

(*a*) *Chlorine*
(*b*) *Hypochlorites* (e.g. Domestos, Chloros)

Wide range of antibacterial activity (except TB). Some spores killed. Rapid action. Greatly inactivated by organic matter. May corrode metals. Cheap. Poor wetting power; addition of **compatible** detergent necessary (as in Thicker Domestos). Non-toxic. Suitable for food preparation areas.

(*c*) *Iodine and iodophors* (e.g. Betadine, Disadine)

Wide range of antibacterial activity. Some spores killed. Rapid action. Some inactivation by organic matter. May corrode metals. Iodophors incorporate detergent. Expensive. Some staining and skin sensitivity.

(*d*) *Formaldehyde gas*

Good disinfectant but difficult to use and unreliable. High humidity and temperature required. Penetration of fabrics poor. Absorbed by rubber.

(*e*) *Formalin solution*

Wide range of activity. Too irritant for routine use. Reserve for instruments contaminated with virus of hepatitis B.

(*f*) *Glutaraldehyde* (e.g. Cidex)

Wide range of activity. Slowly sporicidal. Use only for heat-sensitive instruments which cannot be disinfected any other way (e.g. fibreoptic endoscopes). Poor penetration of organic matter, therefore absolute cleanliness essential before disinfection. Very expensive. Absorbed by rubber and plastics. Toxic and irritant.

4. Quaternary ammonium compounds

(*a*) *Benzalkonium chloride* (e.g. Roccal)
(*b*) *Cetrimide* (e.g. Cetavlon)

Narrow range of antibacterial activity. More active against gram-positives than gram-negatives. Bacteriostatic rather than cidal. Not sporicidal. Inactivated by organic matter and soap. Good detergents. Cheap.

5. Miscellaneous

(a) *Chlorhexidine* (e.g. Hibitane)	Limited range of activity. More active against gram-positives than gram-negatives. Inactivated by organic matter. Not cheap. Useful skin disinfectant.
(b) *Chlorhexidine + Cetrimide* (e.g. Savlon)	As 5 (a). Inactivated by plastic and cellulose. Good detergent. Not cheap.
(c) *Picloxydine + benzalkonium chloride* (e.g. Resiguard)	As 5 (b).

Disinfectants should be used **only** when physical methods are impossible or impracticable or where disposable items cannot be used. For reasons of economy and infection control, disinfectant usage should be minimized by having available a small number of preparations which can be supplied diluted ready for use by the hospital pharmacy. Thus staff can become familiar with their correct use and dilution errors are avoided.

A suitable disinfection policy could incorporate the following:

General disinfection	A phenolic (e.g. Clearsol) incorporating a detergent. Normally used at 0·625%, but in the presence of organic matter (pus, blood, faeces, food) use at 1·0%.
Surface disinfection of 'clean' objects	Hypochlorite 1% with detergent (e.g. Thicker Domestos diluted 1 in 10). Agent of choice for virus of hepatitis B. Where quick drying is required, use industrial methylated spirit (70%).
Handwashing	General wards use plain soap. Theatres and ICU use surgical scrub (e.g. Hibiscrub = chlorhexidine).
Operation sites	Chlorhexidine gluconate 0·5% in 70% spirit.
Wound cleansing	Chlorhexidine + cetrimide (Savlon) diluted 1 in 30 (3%) in sterile water.
Injection or venepuncture	Swabs impregnated with 70% alcohol (e.g. Medi-Swabs).
Instruments contaminated with hepatitis B virus	Formaldehyde solution 1 in 10 (i.e. formalin 10% = formaldehyde 4%).

Equipment

In the intensive care setting, despite environmental considerations, the use of disposable equipment has much to commend it, and where available such items should be chosen. Unfortunately, we are still left with a great mass of machinery which is too expensive to be disposable and which is often very difficult or impossible to sterilize. For non-disposable items, therefore, ease of sterilization should be a major consideration when contemplating their purchase. Only if this is emphasized to manufacturers will they make an effort to produce equipment which can be easily dismantled, cleaned and sterilized.

Ventilators

Many different types of machine are available and used, some of which are extremely difficult to decontaminate and others which have separate, removable and autoclavable patient circuits. Numerous methods have been described for the decontamination of ventilators and they will be only briefly reviewed here.

Ethylene oxide can be used for all types of ventilator. The gas, which is explosive, is mixed with an inert gas such as carbon dioxide and is led from the cylinder to a large plastic bag in which the ventilator is enclosed. The ventilator is switched on and cycled until the circuit is full of gas. The bag is then sealed, left for 24 hours and then evacuated. The ventilator is removed, flushed with air for at least 4 hours and left for a further day or so longer before re-use. Rubber and plastics absorb ethylene oxide and they may require prolonged periods of aeration.

Formaldehyde can be used in one of two ways. In the first, warm, moist formaldehyde is vaporized from the humidifier in a ventilator cycling on closed circuit and recirculated, and in the second the entire machine is enclosed in a special cabinet and cycled in the presence of formaldehyde vapour. As with ethylene oxide, formaldehyde is absorbed by rubber and plastics, and adequate neutralization of the vapour with ammonia followed by aeration is required.

Liquid disinfectants. Some ventilators, which can be cycled on completely closed circuit, may be decontaminated by circulating liquid disinfectants such as Resiguard (*v.s.*) or Savlon (*v.s.*) in water or alcohol. It is a simple and cheap method which washes the internal surfaces of the ventilator clean, but it is sometimes messy and requires considerable work.

Ultrasonic nebulization. Ultrasonic nebulizers are expensive but they have been used to decontaminate ventilators of several types. Nebulized alcohol in nitrogen and hydrogen peroxide have both been used, but because of the risks of explosion with alcohol and failures with hydrogen peroxide this method is now little used.

Autoclavable circuits. A number of ventilators now incorporate separate, removable patient circuits. Their use is preferable to machines which require disinfection but they are costly in capital outlay and in replacements for parts damaged during autoclaving. Nevertheless, auto-claving removes the risk of ventilator-acquired cross-infection.

Bacterial filters. Inspiratory and heated or siliconized expiratory filters can effectively isolate the patient from his ventilator bacteriologically. Thus the ventilator cannot infect the patient and the patient cannot contaminate the ventilator. In these circumstances disinfection of ventilators becomes un-necessary, and the number of ventilators in service in any unit at any time can be doubled by doing away with the need to keep ventilators out of service for disinfection and subsequent airing out.

Humidifiers

These should be autoclavable and of the hot-water type. During use bacterial growth can be prevented by maintaining a temperature of 50° C or above and by keeping the humidifier filled with 0·02% chlorhexidine gluconate in sterile water. As chlorhexidine is virtually non-volatile the humidifier should be topped-up with sterile water, but it should be autoclaved and refilled with 0·02% chlorhexidine gluconate weekly or between patients.

Nebulizers

These are more likely to be a source of infection than hot-water humidifiers because a contaminated nebulizer will blow an aerosol of bacteria-laden droplets into the patient. For this reason they should be avoided, but if they must be used, nebulizer, water-traps and tubing should be sterilized and changed daily. Small-volume nebulizers for specific medicaments are not quite so hazardous but only sterile solutions should be used and removable parts must be sterilized between doses.

Tubing (between ventilator and patient)

Either disposable or sterilizable tubing should be used and changed daily. This manoeuvre reduces the multiplication of potential pathogens and consequently the bacterial challenge to the patient's upper respiratory tract.

Tracheostomy

Patients with recently performed tracheostomies, or endotracheal tubes *in situ*, are extremely susceptible to hospital-acquired pulmonary infections, especially with gram-negative organisms such as *P. aeruginosa*.

A number of mechanisms interact to increase susceptibility to infection. Nasopharyngeal defences are bypassed. Tracheostomy or intubation are frequently required because of the presence of mechanical or physiological pulmonary abnormalities which in themselves increase susceptibility to infection. Furthermore, inhalation therapy and tracheal suction are common routes for the introduction of pathogenic micro-organisms.

Tracheostomy should be performed electively and aseptically in the operating theatre. Emergency tracheostomy may usually be avoided by temporary endotracheal intubation and an elective procedure can follow later. Careful attention to the postoperative wound site is important. All manipulations at the site should be carried out aseptically and gloves should be worn. The skin around the wound should be cleaned with an antibacterial preparation every 8–12 hours. Savlon 3% aqueous (Savlon Liquid Antiseptic) applied with a sterile gauze swab is ideal for this purpose. The wound is dried with another sterile swab, povidone-iodine powder (Disadine Dry Powder spray) applied and then finally covered with a sterile dry dressing. The tracheostomy tube should be changed regularly, under sterile conditions, using a sterile replacement.

A high humidity must be maintained in the tracheobronchial tree, especially in patients recently intubated or tracheostomized. Dry air leads rapidly to desication of the respiratory mucosa, crust formation and the inspissation of secretions, and dry oxygen will inhibit ciliary function. Therefore, inspired air should be completely saturated with moisture and reach the patient at body temperature, necessitating the use of a humidifier or nebulizer.

Inspired air should be sterile, which means that scrupulous attention must be paid to the cleanliness of the humidification apparatus, patient tubing and ventilator (see 'Equipment', above).

Equipment and medicaments used in the care of the intubated or tracheostomized patient must be reserved for that patient only and not shared with other patients. Water and medicaments must be sterile, and solutions should be dispensed from single-dose vials.

A number of workers have demonstrated the effectiveness of, and now routinely use, endotracheal antibiotics locally for the prevention of infection. Valuable therapeutic agents such as gentamicin should not be used prophylactically because of the real danger of gentamicin-resistant organisms, and a combination of two of the less commonly used and less valuable systemic antibiotics—polymyxin B and kanamycin—is particularly suitable. The dosages are: kanamycin 250 mg + polymyxin B 100 000 i.u. (from vials for injection) dissolved in 10 ml isotonic saline, eight-hourly. To administer the treatment a plastic cathether is introduced deeply into the trachea and the antibiotic mixture injected slowly. The three daily doses are given with the patient lying in a different position each time: (1) left lateral, (2) right lateral, and (3) dorsal decubitus position.

Minimizing retained secretions is extremely important in preventing infection since these are an excellent culture medium for the multiplication of potential pathogens. Suction should be performed regularly and as required, aseptically and atraumatically. A fresh sterile catheter must be used every time and then discarded or cleaned and resterilized.

Suction bottles should be changed every 12 hours. After use they should be thoroughly cleaned and sterilized prior to re-use. Portable suction machines require an efficient exhaust filter to prevent the spread of aerosols of bacteria from the vacuum pump.

Venepuncture and intravenous infusion

Venepuncture is an invasive procedure which offers ample opportunity for the introduction of micro-organisms to the blood stream. Intravenous infusions prolong this hazard as there is inevitably some 'in and out' movement of the cannula or catheter at the venepuncture site and manipulations of the venous line provide further opportunities for the introduction of infection. As veins are of vital importance to seriously ill patients, every care must be taken to conserve them; the number of venepunctures should be minimized and cut-downs avoided. Venepunctures and the insertion of venous lines, and all manipulations of them, must be regarded as aseptic procedures and this is particularly important if the line is to be maintained *in situ* for extended periods.

Venepuncture and insertion of intravenous line

The hands must be washed and sterile gloves worn. The skin is prepared by the application of 0·5% chlorhexidine in 70% alcohol (or 70% isopropyl alcohol in an impregnated swab, e.g. Medi-Swab) to a wide area around the venepuncture site, and allowed to dry completely.

Plastic cannulae and catheters should be avoided where possible and metal cannulae (e.g. Butterfly) should be used in preference for peripheral venous lines. After insertion, the cannula is securely taped in place with sterile adhesive tape. The puncture site and the junction with the giving set are sprayed with povidone-iodine powder (Disadine Dry Powder spray) and a dry dressing applied and covered with 3 inch (7·5 cm) elastic strapping. Central venous lines are inserted with similar precautions.

Maintenance of venous lines

If a peripheral venous line has to be maintained over a long period of time it should prove more economical in terms of veins to change the site at least every 48 hours. This will minimize the incidence of phlebitis and preserve the veins for subsequent use.

The administration set should be changed, aseptically, every 24 hours. At this time the dressing over the puncture site should be changed and povidone-iodine powder again applied to the site and to the junction between the cannula and administration set.

If drugs are to be administered intermittently by infusion an administration set with a side-arm should be used. Injections can be made into the side-arm (after swabbing with alcohol) and this avoids disturbing the terminal injection site and dressings on the giving set. If drugs are to be given by intermittent rapid infusion (ideal for i.v. antibiotics) a paediatric burette should be used. It is often possible to 'unblock' a blocked intravenous line by injection into the side-arm without disturbing the dressings at the puncture site.

The effects of drugs which cause phlebitis can usually be minimized by rapid injection into the side-arm followed by 'flushing through' with the infusion fluid. If an irritant drug has to be given by slow infusion, the addition of heparin (2 i.u./ml) to the infusion fluid, and to the succeeding bottle, is helpful.

Changing containers of i.v. fluids is an aseptic procedure. Hands must be washed. The diaphragms of **both** old and new containers are swabbed with alcohol (Medi-Swabs) and allowed to dry completely. The administration set is withdrawn cleanly from the old container and inserted into the new one. If there is even a suspicion that the end of the giving set has touched anything unsterile it must be changed.

Infection at venepuncture site

If the venepuncture site appears inflamed or infected, or if fever develops in a patient who has had a venous line *in situ* for some time, a swab of the

puncture site and the cannula or distal part of the catheter (cut off aseptically), in a sterile container, should be sent immediately to the bacteriology laboratory for culture. Blood for culture should also be taken from a
different vein in febrile patients at the same time.

Bacteriological monitoring

The bacteriological examination of specimens which are not clinically
indicated is generally a waste of time and of little value. In the ICU,
however, routine monitoring can be helpful if used sensibly by providing
evidence of microbial colonization which may subsequently lead to infection. Knowledge of the microbial colonization of patients can be of im-
mense help if severe infection occurs and antibiotic therapy has to be
instituted 'blindly'. Sampling of the inanimate environment is of little value
except in the investigation of epidemics of infection.

The following specimens should be cultured routinely:

1. *Tracheal aspirate*: Daily for evidence of colonization or infection.
2. *Tracheostomy wound swab*: Daily.
3. *Catheter urine*: Daily.
4. *Peritoneal dialysis fluid*: Daily.
5. *Wounds and drain sites*: At first dressing; thereafter if infection is
suspected.

Design and ventilation of intensive care units

No one design is ideal for all requirements and many different designs of
ICU have proved satisfactory. These have usually been compromises which
make the best possible use of available space to suit the types of cases and
equipment encountered locally. The subject is too specialized to be covered
in detail here, but a few of the general principles involved are worthy of
discussion.

The unit should be subdivided into cubicles, with two or three beds to
each, for patients who do not require isolation. Single-bedded cubicles are
required for protective isolation and for containment isolation. The space
allocated to each bed should be greater than in a general ward and must be
sufficient to accommodate a large volume of monitoring equipment and a
ventilator and still permit easy access to the patient. The nursing station
should be sited centrally in the unit to give the best possible view of all the
beds.

Ancillary rooms should be separate but integral with the unit. They
should include clean and 'dirty' utility rooms, CSSD store (of adequate
area), equipment store, staff rest rooms, visitors' room, laboratory, bedroom
for resident medical officer, and a seminar room for case discussions and
teaching. A kitchen with a heated (pasteurizing) dishwasher is essential.

Toilet facilities are required at the entrance to the unit (at least for
handwashing) as well as an area for changing outer clothing. Every bed
should have its own washbasin, and heated sink-traps may be helpful in
reducing cross-infection.

The ventilation system is of major importance. It should incorporate heating, cooling and humidification units and provide proper air conditioning, vital for patient and staff comfort alike, and necessary for efficiency. The system must be designed to maintain the ICU at a positive pressure with respect to the rest of the hospital. Within the unit the isolation cubicles should be ventilated separately. Containment isolation requires exhaust ventilation (negative pressure) to ensure that airborne pathogens are not forced into the rest of the unit and protective isolation must be plenum ventilated (positive pressure) so that potential pathogens are not sucked in from the other areas. To maintain two separate types of isolation cubicle for these special situations is uneconomical and will lead to under-use or wrong use of their beds. Dual-purpose isolation cubicles with switchable ventilation (plenum/exhaust) are dangerous because the wrong ventilation option may be chosen for a particular patient. A sensible alternative to this is an isolation room separated from the rest of the unit by a vestibule. The isolation room and the ICU are both plenum ventilated and the vestibule is exhaust ventilated. By this means the ventilation of the isolation cubicle is kept completely separate from that of the rest of the ICU. The doors leading from the cubicle and from the unit into the vestibule are interlocked so that only one can be open at any one time. Air entering the vestibule from either the unit or the cubicle is sucked out by the exhaust ventilation in the vestibule. Thus there can be no mixing of the atmospheres of the cubicle and the unit and there is no way that airborne microbes can be transferred from the isolation cubicle to the unit or in the reverse direction. A washbasin and coathangers should be placed in the vestibule for washing and gowning before entering the cubicle. This design is ideal for both protective and containment isolation.

Clean areas such as the CSSD store and clean utility room should be plenum ventilated, and the dirty areas such as the sluice and WCs should be exhaust ventilated. The whole unit must have its air changed sufficiently frequently (about 10 times per hour) to provide adequate ventilation, without discomfort or draught, together with effective temperature and humidity control.

Antibiotics

The correct use of antibiotics and chemotherapeutic agents is vitally important in the hospital environment. Misuse of potent antimicrobial agents leads not only to an increase in patient morbidity but also to the colonization of the areas where misuse occurs (often the ICU) by highly resistant strains of micro-organisms. The occurrence of resistant strains is generally proportional to the use of any antibiotic, and prophylactic and topical use of antibiotics can aggravate this. The reasons are, at least superficially, simple. If a particular antibiotic is widely used (or misused!) an environmental selective pressure is exerted which confers an advantage on hospital strains of bacteria resistant to that antibiotic and they multiply in that environment. They may also, and often do, pass on their resistances to other bacterial strains and species and this can complicate the problem further. When the selective pressures are removed, possibly by restricting or prohibiting the use of the offending antibiotic and related compounds, the resistant organisms lose their advantage and they are overgrown by other less resistant bacterial strains.

It is thus essential and obvious that every well run establishment should have an antibiotic policy which has been agreed by surgeon, physician, anaesthetist and microbiologist. In common with other policies this will inevitably be a compromise.

Antibiotic policy

Antibiotic prophylaxis

This should be restricted to those patients who require it, and the indications for systemic antibiotic prophylaxis are relatively few. If broad spectrum antibiotics, such as the cephalosporins, ampicillin and gentamicin, are used indiscriminately resistant organisms will be selected, will spread and will cause infection. This has been well described in a number of outbreaks where the problem was solved only when antibiotics were withdrawn entirely for a period of time and subsequently used only where clinically and microbiologically indicated.

Where systemic antibiotic prophylaxis is indicated a **narrow spectrum** agent (or combination of agents) should be chosen which is directly **specifically** against the small group of potential pathogens which are liable to cause trouble in that situation. Broad spectrum prophylaxis must be avoided because of its profound effect on the normally sensitive body microflora which will be replaced by hospital strains of multiple-resistant pathogens. The longer the period during which antibiotic prophylaxis is given before operation, the more profound is the disturbance of normal body flora and the greater is the opportunity for colonization with hospital pathogens.

Thus prophylactic regimens should not be started until immediately before operation (e.g. with the premedication drugs). They should incorporate only narrow spectrum drugs aimed at specific bacteria, and they should be given for only a short time postoperatively.

The main indications for antibiotic prophylaxis and suitable antibacterial agents are as follows:

Lower limb amputation for peripheral vascular diseases. Give penicillin (erythromycin in allergic patients) to prevent gas gangrene caused by *Clostridium welchii* which is present in the rectum and on the buttocks of all patients.

Open-heart surgery. The main risk is of postoperative endocarditis caused by *Staphylococcus epidermidis* or diphtheroids from the skin of the patient or surgeon. Cloxacillin combined with vancomycin (or the less specific streptomycin) provides adequate cover and prophylaxis should be started with premedication and continued for no longer than 72 hours postoperatively. If continued longer, there is a danger of infection with Candida.

Upper abdominal surgery on chronic bronchitics. Postoperative chest infections in these patients may be reduced by the use of ampicillin. It should not be used for operations on other sites or on non-bronchitic patients.

Neurosurgery. Some types of neurosurgery merit similar prophylaxis to that given for open-heart surgery (*v.s.*)

Restriction of antibiotic usage

Some antibiotics should not be used in hospital (with minor exceptions) and others should be reserved for clearly defined indications, leaving only a few for 'general' use. 'Blind' therapy and combination therapy should be avoided except in severely ill patients with clinical signs of infection (e.g. septic shock). Where possible, infections should be treated only with the specific agents listed in bacteriological sensitivity reports.

Tetracyclines should be avoided, as should ampicillin (and amoxycillin) except in acute exacerbations of chronic bronchitis and in urinary tract infections. The aminoglycoside antibiotics (gentamicin, tobramycin and kanamycin), the cephalosporins and carbenicillin should be reserved for severe infections and prescribed on the basis of bacterial sensitivity reports.

Gentamicin and the cephalosporins are potentially nephrotoxic when used together and this combination is to be avoided. Cephalosporins (particularly cephaloridine) should not be used when the patient is receiving diuretic therapy (especially with frusemide) as there is a real danger of acute renal failure.

Treatment of infection

The treatment of infection is a vast subject which cannot be covered in detail here. Where clinical circumstances permit, the commencement of antibiotic therapy should be delayed until bacterial sensitivities and resistances are known. Therapy can then be commenced with the appropriate agent specific for that infection and the dangers of superinfection minimized.

The major pathogens in hospital often have predictable sensitivities which are outlined in Table 15.2.

Some patients who present with clinical signs of severe infection, such as septic shock or pneumonia, require initial (blind) antibiotic therapy. In these cases the delay in waiting for culture and sensitivity results may be fatal. Therefore therapy with an empirical combination of antibiotics is commenced as soon as all appropriate specimens (blood cultures, swabs, sputum, urine) have been taken for bacteriological culture. A suitable combination is gentamicin (6 mg/kg per day) with carbenicillin (500 mg/kg per day) given separately in rapid infusions by the intravenous route. Whatever the patient's renal function is, a full loading dose of each agent should be given—for adults, gentamicin 160 mg + carbenicillin 10 g. Maintenance doses can then be calculated on the basis of creatinine clearance (easily calculated from serum creatinine levels). As soon as sensitivity results are

TABLE 15.2.   SENSITIVITIES OF MAJOR HOSPITAL PATHOGENS

Pathogen	Usually sensitive to*
Staphylococcus aureus	Flucloxacillin, (clindamycin).
Escherichia coli	Co-trimoxazole, gentamicin, (ampicillin), (amoxycillin).
Klebsiella	Cefazolin, (gentamicin), (tobramycin), (amikacin).
Pseudomonas aeruginosa	Gentamicin, carbenicillin, (tobramycin), (amikacin).

* Second choice agents are in parentheses.

available, specific therapy can be commenced and antibiotics can be added to or deleted from the initial regimen. Failure to do this will lead to super-infection with multiple-resistant bacteria or Candida.

Conclusion

Patients requiring tracheostomy and ventilation need intensive care and they are peculiarly liable to infection. The bacteriological problems in intensive care units are many and complex, and it is only by good team work and strict adherence to agreed policies for the control of infection and antibiotic usage that the dangers can be minimized.

Chapter 16

Intensive Care in a District General Hospital

The aim of intensive care, irrespective of the type of hospital concerned, is to give the best available specialized vital support to the critically ill patient to ensure his ultimate recovery. Nevertheless, the inherent differences of staffing, facilities, resources and the specialized nature of the diseases referred for treatment in teaching institutions must influence the character and function of their intensive care units. District general hospitals, which provide the majority of patient care in the United Kingdom, tend to treat a wider and more representative cross-section of disease. In teaching hospitals several separate therapy units may coexist, each with its own specialized nursing and medical staffs. District general hospitals are likely to afford the resources and staff for only one or two specialized units. In teaching hospitals the severity and heroic nature of the surgery practised implies the need for complementary postoperative care which cannot be carried out in the general wards; in a district hospital, it is usually the severity of the patient's primary illness that demands intensive care rather than the effects of a surgical operation.

This chapter describes the experience of an intensive care unit in the district general hospital at Kingston-upon-Thames during the nine years from 1967 to 1975. It makes no claim to represent the unit as an ideal or a model which others should emulate; its only claim is that the unit has attempted to meet the needs of the patients who have been admitted and the demands of the clinicians who have treated them. From the start it was clear that, in spite of preconceived ideas as to how such a unit should be managed, it was found possible to do so only by a consensus of those who had to treat patients in it. Thus the management policy of any intensive care unit becomes tailored to a compromise between the pressures and strains of sometimes irreconcilable therapeutic opinions.

Before establishing the unit the fundamental decision had to be taken as to whether or not patients requiring coronary care should be admitted to the same unit as those requiring other forms of intensive care. At the outset prevailing opinion was heavily against the suggestion. Patients with myocardial infarction need privacy and quietude and should not be disturbed by the noise associated with patients requiring heavy nursing, respiratory care and treatment for drug overdose. On the other hand, this district general hospital was unable to afford two special care units. It was found in practice that the intake of coronary care patients has been fairly constant

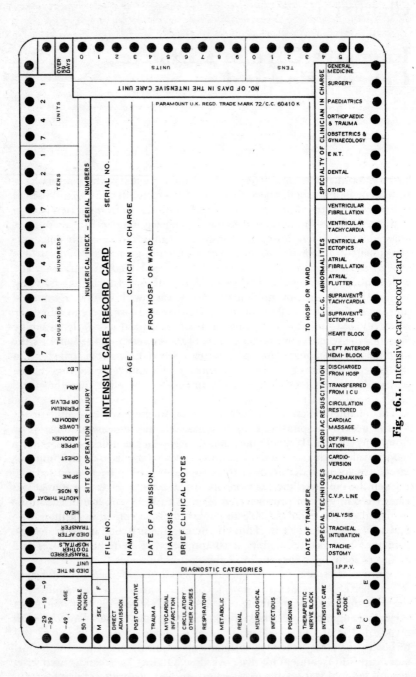

Fig. 16.1. Intensive care record card.

and has justified the retention of special nursing staff against the variable demands of the unit for other forms of intensive care. A unit that excluded 'coronaries' would occasionally find itself fully staffed by nurses with no patients to care for. Thus a compromise solution was found whereby patients with myocardial infarction were treated in five single rooms while patients requiring other forms of care were accommodated in an open four-bedded ward. On many occasions the flexibility of the unit was demonstrated when isolation in a single cubicle was required for an intensive care patient or a superfluity of coronary care patients demanded the temporary use of a bed in the open ward.

Because a district general hospital serves all the needs of the local community the changing nature of the patients treated in its intensive care unit reflects the changing trends of serious disease in the population and the popularity of certain forms of therapy. The changes in the nature of the underlying diseases that caused the patients' admission to the intensive care unit and the types of treatment instituted over the years from 1967 to 1975 are presented in this chapter to give an indication of the trends that have been observed in this community hospital.

The unit at Kingston Hospital has nine beds and provides intensive nursing facilities in addition to the life support functions of an intensive therapy unit. Although patients with a very wide range of diseases of varying severity have been admitted, a policy has been adopted of returning the patients to the general ward as soon as their condition was considered to be suitable for general ward nursing. These decisions were made by the clinician under whose care the patient was admitted although the ultimate over-all responsibility for the management of the unit remained under the supervision of an anaesthetist.

At an early stage it was decided to attempt to limit the number of patients in the intensive care unit according to the availability of trained nursing staff. The sister-in-charge was allowed to exercise discretion as to how many beds of the maximum total of nine she could cover adequately; to spread the highly specialized staff too thinly in this area of peak nursing demand was considered to be bad practice.

From the time that the unit was opened in 1966, records of each patient admitted were kept on a punch card (Fig. 16.1) and the function of the unit was regularly surveyed in a Report published each year. In this chapter the details of the work of the unit and the changing trends in the need for therapy are presented against the background of these Annual Reports published from 1967 to 1975.

Statistical summary of admissions to the intensive care unit, Kingston Hospital, 1967–75

Intensive care patients

The 7 039 admissions to the unit from 1967 to 1975 are separated into three categories and, as might be expected, 80% were recorded as 'intensive care' (Table 16.1). The scope of this term has widened from the

TABLE 16.1.   ADMISSIONS TO THE INTENSIVE CARE UNIT,
KINGSTON HOSPITAL, 1967–75

Total patients admitted		7 039
Intensive care patients		5 624
Direct admissions to the unit	3 959	
Transfers from other wards or		
from other hospitals in the area	1 665	
Short-stay patients		1 104
Pain clinic patients		311

original narrow definition of intensive care as implying moment to moment medical and nursing care of a patient requiring mechanical support to life. Intensive care at Kingston Hospital is broadly defined as the treatment of patients likely to benefit from the special nursing, monitoring and therapeutic facilities of the Unit, having regard to the conditions prevailing in the general wards of the hospital. It is theoretically possible to imagine a hospital so lavishly staffed and equipped that an intensive care unit would be superfluous. At the other end of the scale a hospital might be so short of nurses, doctors and equipment, that all seriously ill patients would pass through one favoured ward known as the intensive care unit. Thus every individual hospital finds itself somewhere between the two extremes and must use its intensive care facilities not according to a doctrinaire policy but in accordance with the best interests of all its patients.

The overwhelming majority of medical patients were direct admissions; this implies that beds had to be found for them in the general wards when they were fit for transfer from the Unit. By contrast, the majority of the surgical patients already had their beds allocated, the severity of the operation being the usual reason for their requiring intensive care. Surgical cases arriving as direct admissions to the Unit were usually emergencies from the operating theatre and those with accidental injuries.

Short-stay patients

It has always been considered unrealistic and unhelpful to lay down rigid criteria for admission to the Unit. As a result, many patients were admitted as a precaution against their deterioration in contrast to those who had already proved their need for intensive care in the general wards or before admission to hospital. Thus the intensive care category refers only to those whose illness, viewed in retrospect, required the special facilities of the Unit. The patients who, with hindsight, could have been treated equally satisfactorily in the ordinary wards of the hospital were included in the 'short-stay' category. For instance, as the mortality from myocardial infarction is highest in the first 24 hours following admission it was thought better to admit all patients with precordial pain direct to the Unit, investigate and monitor them overnight, and then to move them the following day if the diagnosis of myocardial infarction was unconfirmed and the special precautions were not justified.

Pain clinic patients

No formal pain clinic was established at the hospital but owing to the lack of facilities elsewhere it was found convenient to see patients with intractable pain in the Intensive Care Unit. Until 1974, when alternative accommodation was found, 311 patients had been given nerve blocks for cancer pain or for acute and chronic lumbosciatic pain.

Intensive care patients: distribution by diagnosis

TABLE 16.2. DISTRIBUTION BY DIAGNOSIS: INTENSIVE CARE PATIENTS

	1967–69	1970–72	1973–75	Totals 1967–75	Over-all Mortality
Postoperative	288 (37)	283 (31)	301 (39)	872 (107)	12·2%
Trauma	114 (19)	89 (20)	85 (9)	288 (48)	16·7%
Myocardial infarction	672 (98)	873 (112)	830 (105)	2 375 (315)	13·3%
Other circulatory disease	161 (24)	167 (18)	356 (33)	684 (75)	11·0%
Respiratory disease	155 (27)	78 (24)	91 (25)	324 (76)	23·4%
Metabolic disease	9 (2)	9 (2)	18	36 (4)	11·1%
Renal disease	15 (2)	24 (10)	21 (2)	60 (14)	23·3%
Neurological disease	57 (20)	36 (19)	61 (36)	154 (75)	48·7%
Infectious disease	—	10 (3)	21 (8)	31 (11)	35·5%
Poisoning	252 (8)	288 (7)	255 (3)	795 (18)	2·3%
Others	2 (2)	1 (1)	2	5 (3)	—
Totals	1 725 (239)	1 858 (247)	2 041 (260)	5 624 (746)	13·3%

Figures in parentheses indicate deaths.

Table 16.2 gives a general impression of the frequency with which various types of disease required intensive care. Postoperative patients included 427 following thoracotomy for oesophageal and lung surgery, together with 111 others who required temporary artificial ventilation. Admissions for the care of serious injuries were unexpectedly low, averaging only 32 per year; the majority were patients unconscious with head injury following road traffic accidents. The postoperative and traumatic categories, i.e. surgical patients, accounted for only 21% of admissions.

Patients with myocardial infarction comprised 42% of all admissions. These, together with patients suffering from other circulatory disease, occupied the monitored beds in the coronary care section of the Unit to an increasing extent over the 9 years. Thus 'circulatory care' patients accounted for 48% of admissions in 1967–69, increasing to 58% in 1973–75.

The need for the admission of patients with respiratory disease has diminished in recent years; certainly the numbers of patients with chronic obstructive lung disease requiring long-term artificial ventilation (IPPV) in the early years of the Unit were rarely seen in more recent times.

Sixty patients with renal failure were admitted for peritoneal dialysis or for assessment before transfer to special units for haemodialysis.

Patients with neurological disease constituted the group with the highest mortality. Many had suffered a cerebrovascular accident who presented on admission as unconscious with respiratory failure. The diagnosis usually lay between a drug overdose and a cerebrovascular accident but when the latter diagnosis had been confirmed there was no alternative but to continue with the ventilator therapy which had already been started. A few patients recovered to be discharged from hospital but in the rest the irreversibility of brain damage became apparent and treatment was discontinued.

Patients with drug overdose and other poisoning accounted for 14% of admissions; the majority were healthy in all other respects and, in consequence, this group showed by far the lowest mortality.

Special techniques in intensive care

TABLE 16.3.   SPECIAL TECHNIQUES IN INTENSIVE CARE

	1967–69	1970–72	1973–75	Totals
IPPV and tracheostomy	67 ⎱ 232	34 ⎱ 204	20 ⎱ 293	121 ⎱ 729
IPPV and tracheal intubation	165 ⎰	170 ⎰	273 ⎰	608 ⎰
Tracheostomy only	17	21	9	47
Tracheal intubation only	109	150	101	360
External cardiac massage	175	207	175	557
Internal cardiac massage	1	—	1	2
Electrical defibrillation	55	95	88	238
Cardioversion	68	56	90	214
Temporary cardiac pacing	31	18	58	107
Peritoneal dialysis	26	27	20	73
Therapeutic epidural analgesia	2	2	—	4

The special techniques used in intensive care reflect some of the changes in therapy over the past 9 years. Most noticeable is the recent increased use of IPPV via an endotracheal tube in preference to tracheostomy. In explanation, one may point not only to the reduced incidence of respiratory failure in patients with chronic lung disease but also to the availability of suitable non-irritating endotracheal tubes which ensure that it is safe to maintain an airway by this means for several days. The use of tracheostomy without IPPV is now restricted mainly to patients with irremediable upper respiratory obstruction.

While external massage rightly remains the preferred method of cardiac resuscitation, 2 cases of open chest cardiac massage are recorded. The higher frequency of electrical defibrillation, cardioversion and cardiac pacing reflects the increasing use of the coronary care section of the Unit.

During the 6 years 1967–72 the value of temporary cardiac pacing for the treatment of heart block associated with myocardial infarction was well appreciated, but the application of the technique was limited by the fitful local availability of the skill necessary to insert the pacing electrode. For this reason only 49 patients were paced in the unit while 32 were transferred elsewhere for temporary pacing and 7 for the insertion of a permanent pacemaker. From 1973 to 1975, and coincidentally with the acquisition of an image intensifier, 58 patients were paced in the Unit; there were no transfers for temporary pacing but 17 patients were sent to specialized units for insertion of permanent pacemakers.

Coronary care in the intensive care unit

The patients treated for myocardial infarction were nursed in five separate cubicles each with an individual heart rate monitor and oscilloscope. This was linked at the nurses' station with a multi-channel oscilloscope screen, automatic alarm and ECG write-out. The nurses were trained to recognize serious arrhythmias and, in the absence of a doctor, to administer intravenous lignocaine and to carry out cardiac massage, defibrillation, tracheal intubation and oxygenation.

Table 16.4 shows the increasing incidence of admissions for myocardial

TABLE 16.4. MYOCARDIAL INFARCTION: ADMISSIONS AND BED OCCUPANCY

	1967–69	1970–72	1973–75	Totals
Patients admitted	672 (98)	873 (112)	830 (105)	2 375 (315)
Mortality	14·6%	12·8%	12·6%	13·3%
Bed occupancy in patient-days	2 507	2 675	2 174	7 356
Days per patient	3·7	3·1	2·6	3·1

Figures in parentheses indicate deaths.

infarction over the years under review, with a substantially constant mortality rate, but with a shorter average period of bed occupancy per patient. Comparing 1973–75 with 1967–69, 158 more patients were treated in 333 fewer patient-days.

TABLE 16.5. MYOCARDIAL INFARCTION:
MORTALITY AND LENGTH OF STAY

Days in the Unit	Patients	Deaths
1	511	202
2	712	43
3	517	19
4	253	8
5	145	11
6	74	7
7	60	6
8	31	3
9	23	4
10 and over	49	12
Totals	2 375	315

It is well recognized that patients are at the greatest risk of cardiac arrest during the first 24–48 hours from the onset of symptoms. Table 16.5 shows that 64% of the deaths occurred on the first day in the Unit, 78% in the first two days and 84% in the first three days following admission. It was therefore assumed that the majority of patients could, with reasonable safety, be transferred to the general medical wards after a stay of two days. A longer stay in the Unit was indicated after resuscitation from cardiac arrest and for those with persistent pain, circulatory failure or arrhythmias.

The longest stay patients were those treated for heart block by transvenous pacemaking. Thus to transfer any patient from the Unit involved taking a calculated risk based on clinical judgement and experience; unfortunately, figures are not available of the number of 'late deaths' occurring in the general wards.

During the years 1973–75 there was a marked trend towards the earlier transfer of patients from the Unit (Table 16.6). This was not entirely due to the increased confidence of the clinicians in selecting those whose safety would not thereby be jeopardized; one must also take into account the exceptional demand on the five coronary care beds for other serious circulatory disease and the recurring episodes of severe shortage of trained nursing staff that inevitably curtailed bed occupancy.

Table 16.6 shows the recent trend towards earlier transfer of patients to

TABLE 16.6. CHANGE OF POLICY IN TRANSFERRING NON-FATAL CASES FROM THE CORONARY CARE UNIT

Patients transferred after	1967–69	1970–72	1973–75
1st day	9%	9%	26%
2nd day	39%	45%	58%
3rd day	62%	70%	81%
4th day	77%	84%	89%
5th day	85%	91%	94%

the general wards. In particular, as many as 26% spent only one day in the unit in 1973–75 in contrast to 9% in earlier years.

Age, sex and mortality

The patients admitted to the Unit for the treatment of myocardial infarction reflect the well recognized relationship of age and sex with the incidence and mortality of the disease.

Table 16.7 shows that the peak incidence was in the sixties in both sexes, the disease being, over all, four times more common and tending to occur at an earlier age in males than in females. The mortality for either sex was similar in all the age groups and increased with advancing age. The ratio of male to female patients was 10:1 in the three decades from 20 to 50, 5:1 in the fifties, 3:1 in the sixties and 2:1 in the seventies.

Interpretation of the results of treatment of myocardial infarction

One cannot draw accurate conclusions concerning the over-all mortality of myocardial infarction and the efficacy of treatment in the coronary care unit. The crude mortality was 315 out of 2 375, or 13·3% of all admissions. Many patients died before admission, some in the ambulance, some in the casualty department and some were moribund on arrival in the Unit. It is not known whether more rapid transport to the hospital would have

TABLE 16.7   MYOCARDIAL INFARCTION: AGE, SEX AND MORTALITY

Age (years)	Males	Females	Totals
20–29	8	1	9
30–39	52(2) *4%*	5(1) —	57(3) *5%*
40–49	307(23) *7%*	31(2) *6%*	338(25) *7%*
50–59	636(67) *11%*	123(12) *10%*	759(79) *10%*
60–69	710(107) *15%*	228(33) *14%*	938(140) *15%*
70–79	169(39) *23%*	82(21) *26%*	251(60) *24%*
80–89	17(5) *29%*	6(3) —	23(8) *35%*
Totals	1 899(243) *13%*	476(72) *15%*	2 375(315) *13%*

Figures in parentheses indicate deaths.

resulted in a saving of lives or in an apparent increase in the Unit's mortality figures. It is known, however, that a number of patients died in the general wards following transfer from the Unit. Others died in the Unit following readmission from the general ward; thus each patient would count as two admissions but only one death. It is estimated that the corrected hospital mortality for all patients admitted to the Unit was about 18%. Caution is therefore needed when comparing mortality rates in different coronary care units. One must take into account not only the speed with which patients are admitted following the onset of symptoms but also the varying local criteria justifying a definitive diagnosis of myocardial infarction.

The main purpose of a coronary care unit is to prevent cardiac arrest by the early detection and intensive treatment of arrhythmias. If cardiac arrest occurs then it must be treated promptly and efficiently. In this Unit, from 1967 to 1975, resuscitation from cardiac arrest was attempted in 344 patients with myocardial infarction, of whom 55 left the hospital alive. These are the only hard facts that can be adduced to justify specialized coronary care; the number of patients in whom cardiac arrest was prevented will always remain a matter for surmise.

Results of cardiac resuscitation

Table 16.8 shows the results of cardiac resuscitation in 559 patients. The frequency with which spontaneous circulation could be restored was 308/559—55%. Many of these patients succumbed to subsequent arrests from which resuscitation became progressively more difficult to achieve as the cardiac output remained inadequate to maintain life. Thus only 120 (39%) of the 308 patients surviving the initial arrest recovered sufficiently to enable them to be transferred to the general wards. Of these 120, only 79 (66%) survived to be discharged from hospital. Hence, the ultimate recovery rate of all patients in whom cardiac resuscitation was attempted was 79 out of 559 or 14%.

TABLE 16.8.   RESULTS OF CARDIAC RESUSCITATION

	Resuscitation attempted	Circulation restored	Transferred from intensive care	Discharged from hospital	Ultimate recovery rate
Myocardial infarction	344	187	78	55	16%
Other cases	215	121	42	24	11%
Totals	559	308	120	79	14%

Attempted resuscitation in patients with myocardial infarction resulted in an ultimate success rate of 16%. Of the 55 survivors, 13 had transvenous pacemaking for heart block and among the remainder the resuscitative measures had almost invariably included direct current defibrillation.

Respiratory intensive care

The special care of patients treated with intermittent positive pressure ventilation (IPPV) is the chief single purpose of intensive care units and originally was the main justification for their establishment. It is the function above all that satisfies the original definition of intensive care, namely the provision of temporary mechanical support of life.

TABLE 16.9.   THE FLUCTUATIONS AND TRENDS IN THE USE OF IPPV 1967–75

	1967	1968	1969	1970	1971	1972	1973	1974	1975
Ventilator-days	621	417	259	210	191	229	206	237	277
Patients ventilated	70	90	72	62	62	80	185	102	106
Average days per patient	8·9	4·6	3·6	3·4	3·1	2·9	2·4	2·3	2·6
Maximum number of ventilators in use on any one day	7	4	4	3	4	3	3	4	3
Days in the year on which 3 or more ventilators were required	82	43	6	7	5	6	4	5	11
Days in the year on which no patient was on IPPV	78	114	171	186	222	187	205	180	178

Over the course of 9 years, the frequency of use of IPPV has fluctuated and its indications have changed. Table 16.9 shows that the annual total of ventilator-days fell from 621 in 1967 to an average of 240 for 1973–75. The average number of days on IPPV per patient was reduced from 8·9 in 1967 to 2·5 in 1973–75. This is almost certainly due to a reduction in the number of patients ventilated on a long-term basis for chronic respiratory disease.

The year 1971 is seen as the lowest for the use of IPPV with only 62 patients ventilated, on 191 ventilator-days; on 222 days in the year no ventilator was in use. More recently there was an increased frequency of ventilator usage and in 1975 no less than 106 patients were ventilated but mostly for a very short period.

In 1967 as many as 7 ventilators were in use on one day but in succeeding years no more than 3 or 4 ventilators were ever in use at the same time. In 1967 there were 82 days on which 3 or more ventilators were simultaneously in use but from 1969–1975 this number was required on relatively few occasions.

Indications for intermittent positive pressure ventilation

TABLE 16.10.   SUMMARY OF INDICATIONS FOR IPPV

	1967–69	1070–72	1073–75	Totals	Mortality
Post-operative respiratory insufficiency	22(7)	25(6)	64(21)	111(34)	31%
Head injury	10(10)	8(7)	7(5)	25(22)	88%
Fractured ribs	5(2)	7(2)	8(2)	20(6)	30%
Following resuscitation from cardiac arrest	53(46)	49(39)	107(81)	209(166)	79%
Other circulatory diseases	3(2)	4(2)	1(1)	8(5)	—
Chronic obstructive chest disease	46(12)	26(14)	15(5)	87(31)	36%
Pneumonia	9(5)	12(8)	6(4)	27(17)	63%
Status asthmaticus	7(2)	5	7(2)	19(4)	21%
Other respiratory diseases	10(3)	3	2(1)	15(4)	—
Cerebrovascular accident	13(11)	11(9)	27(27)	51(47)	92%
Miscellaneous neurological conditions	4(2)	8(7)	4(3)	16(12)	—
Infections	—	—	3(1)	3(1)	—
Poisoning	50(7)	46(5)	42(3)	138(15)	11%
Totals	232(109)	204(99)	293(156)	729(364)	50%

Figures in parentheses indicate deaths.

Mechanical artificial ventilation was carried out on 729 patients or 13% of all patients admitted for intensive care. Table 16.10 summarizes all the indications for IPPV over the nine years under review, together with the attendant mortality for each indication.

The largest group (209 patients) were those following resuscitation from cardiac arrest. There has been a growing conviction in recent years that temporary elective ventilation may marginally improve the chances of ultimate recovery in a group with an admittedly high mortality.

There were 138 patients ventilated following drug poisoning; this represents 17·3% of all patients suffering from poisoning, with an over-all group mortality of 2·3%. There was a mortality of 11% among those who required artificial ventilation, many of whom had suffered severe cerebral hypoxia with irreversible brain damage before admission. No change in trends can be discerned in this group in the frequency of the need for IPPV in spite of the changing trends in prescribing of drugs.

An increasing number of patients have been ventilated for postoperative respiratory insufficiency due to the elective use of the technique in poor-risk surgical cases in whom wound pain itself or its treatment with narcotic analgesics would risk respiratory failure, and it is felt that many patients might otherwise have been denied surgical treatment. Short-term postoperative ventilation was also carried out on some patients in whom the anaesthetist was unable immediately to restore adequate spontaneous respiration following the use of muscle relaxants.

The over-all mortality of patients requiring IPPV was 50%. However, this figure includes three groups of patients whose prognosis was poor when ventilation was started, namely, those with head injury, those with cerebrovascular accident and those following resuscitation from cardiac arrest. It is these patients whose condition may demand difficult ethical decisions as to when the ventilator should be switched off, and yet the ultimate survival of even a few suggests that the decision should not be taken too hastily.

The groups with a lower mortality included patients with flail chests, with exacerbations of chronic obstructive lung disease, pneumonia with respiratory failure and with status asthmaticus for whom temporary artificial ventilation may be an important and life-saving adjunct to therapy.

The treatment of poisoning

Over 100 different drugs are believed to have been taken by 795 patients admitted for the treatment of poisoning. Many patients had taken more than one drug; Table 16.11 lists those selected for comment either because

TABLE 16.11

	1967–69	1970–72	1973–75	Totals
Hypnotic drugs				
All barbiturates	125	131	92	348
Amylobarbitone (Amytal) ⎫ Amylobarbitone with ⎬ quinalbarbitone (Tuinal) ⎭	57	42	49	148
Unidentified barbiturates	30	49	19	98
Methaqualone and diphenhydramine (Mandrax)	30	34	12	76
Nitrazepam (Mogadon)	1	15	20	36
Psychotropic drugs				
Diazepam (Valium)	11	26	42	79
Chlordiazepoxide (Librium)	26	10	12	48
Phenothiazines	22	17	15	54
All antidepressants	31	44	81	156
Tricyclic antidepressants	29	41	77	147
Miscellaneous poisons				
Aspirin, paracetamol and other oral analgesic drugs	37	54	60	151
Alcohol	18	26	22	66
Carbon monoxide	5	6	—	11

of the frequency with which they were implicated or because of a changing trend in their use for attempted suicide over the years under review.

Comment

In the nine years reviewed, 795 patients were admitted for the intensive therapy of poisoning of whom 18 died. Among the drugs taken, barbiturates figured most commonly; significant levels were found in the blood of half the patients admitted in 1967–69 though this proportion dropped to one-third in 1973–75. By far the commonest barbiturate taken appeared to be amylobarbitone (Amytal) alone or in its combination with quinalbarbitone (Tuinal). In about a quarter of the patients with barbiturate poisoning the identity of the particular drug could not be determined.

Among other hypnotics, the most frequently implicated in 1967–69 was methaqualone with diphenhydramine (Mandrax), which was originally introduced as a 'safe' hypnotic. Its safety has subsequently been questioned, and certainly when taken in overdose it has posed difficult problems in treatment including 2 patients who required tracheostomy. It was, however, implicated in only 2 of the 18 poisoning fatalities in the Unit. The apparent recent decline in its use has been matched by an increase in the number of patients admitted with overdoses of nitrazepam (Mogadon) and diazepam (Valium).

An increasing number of patients appeared to have taken drugs used for the treatment of pathological depression; nearly all the drugs implicated belonged to the tricyclic series while mono-amine oxidase inhibitors had been taken by only five patients. Among the less specific psychotropic drugs, chlordiazepoxide (Librium) and the phenothiazines figure less frequently in recent years than formerly.

The narcotics controlled under the Dangerous Drugs Act 1965 have been taken by only 12 patients. At first sight this might be seen as evidence of effective control over their use, but the difficulty of identification by the laboratory must also be considered, particularly when taken in association with other drugs. In any case, when obtained illegally, they are likely to be used more for self-gratification than as a means of attempted suicide.

Among the oral analgesics taken the commonest were aspirin and paracetamol, either by themselves or compounded with similar substances most of which are available to the public without prescription. This group accounted for 7 of the 18 fatal cases.

There remain for consideration a miscellaneous group of poisons. Alcohol levels were found in 66 patients, usually in combination with other drugs. With the advent of natural gas in the district in 1971, it is not surprising that only 11 patients were found to have inhaled detectable amounts of carbon monoxide. Three patients suffered from iatrogenic poisoning, 1 with digoxin and 2 with warfarin.

It is of some interest to note the age and sex distribution of patients admitted for the treatment of poisoning (Table 16.12). While females outnumber males in the proportion of 7 to 4, it should be noted that the most striking sex difference occurred in the sixties. The twenties was the

TABLE 16.12   AGE AND SEX OF PATIENTS ADMITTED
FOR THE TREATMENT OF POISONING, 1967–75

Age (years)	Male	Female	Totals
0– 9	1	5	6
10–19	31	51	82
20–29	101	130	231
30–39	46	98	144
40–49	47	83	130
50–59	37	77	114
60–69	14	44	58
70–79	7	13	20
80–89	4	5	9
90–99	1	—	1
	289	506	795

commonest group for both sexes, in which males approached nearest to parity with females, but from the thirties onwards females were preponderant.

Respiratory support was required in 32·1% of patients and IPPV in 17·4%. Six patients required tracheostomy, a procedure to be avoided if possible, not only for the more obvious reasons but also because the scar is a permanent reminder of an unhappy episode best forgotten. Tracheostomy

TABLE 16.13.   RESPIRATORY SUPPORT IN PATIENTS ADMITTED WITH POISONING, 1967–75

	1967–69	1970–72	1973–75	Totals
Total cases	252	288	255	795
IPPV tracheostomy	2	—	1	3
IPPV tube	48	46	41	135
Tracheostomy only	1	1	1	3
Intubation only	42	38	34	114
Total requiring respiratory support	93 (36·9%)	85 (29·5%)	77 (30·2%)	255 (32·1%)

was carried out with reluctance because of prolonged unconsciousness and difficulty in maintaining adequate tracheobronchial suction through a tracheal tube.

While the figures cannot be cited as indicating a reduction in the need for IPPV, they do suggest a small but significant reduction in the need for over-all respiratory support in the years 1970–75 as compared with 1967–69.

Comment

A change in the prescribing habits of doctors is likely to be the main factor in the changing identity of drugs taken in overdose. It is not believed that patients are particularly discriminating when attempting suicide; they presumably take the drugs which happen to be at hand.

It is also difficult to draw many other conclusions concerning poisoning and its treatment from the statistics relating to patients admitted to the Unit. They are necessarily a selected group, having survived long enough to be admitted alive and yet having impressed the admitting doctor sufficiently with the gravity of their condition to warrant his choosing the Intensive Care Unit for their treatment in preference to the general ward.

One hopes that all patients likely to benefit from intensive care were admitted to the Unit, although a few must have suffered such a degree of cerebral hypoxia as to preclude the possibility of complete recovery. Yet even in these cases there is little alternative to taking the hint from Tennyson's lines:

'No life that breathes with human breath
Has ever truly longed for death.'

Nursing staffing in the intensive care unit

It is well appreciated that the success of an intensive care unit depends primarily on a cadre of nurses trained to understand the intricacies of complex therapy and competent to take the initiative in emergency treatment—abilities which might otherwise be expected of medically qualified personnel. The history of this Unit has been characterized by the constant effort made to maintain these high standards against the background of recurring nursing shortage.

TABLE 16.14.   VARIABILITY IN NURSING STAFFING IN THE INTENSIVE CARE UNIT

	1967	1970	1975
Nurses trained in intensive care	12	4	10 (including 4 agency nurses)
Registered nurses training in intensive care	—	12	8
Enrolled nurses	2	—	4
Student nurses	7	7	4
Totals	21	23	26

The initial enthusiasm with which the Unit opened in 1966 produced a stable team of sisters and staff nurses who together gradually gathered the knowledge and expertise to practise intensive care with a high degree of efficiency. Staffing changes were few and morale was high, so that by the end of 1967 the Unit could boast 12 nurses locally trained in intensive care out of a total staff of 21 (Table 16.14). Then marriage took its toll of the trained staff and their replacement proved impossible. The only solution was to attract nurses from elsewhere by offering an organized six-months course of instruction in intensive care in the hope that some would remain as permanencies. Thus, by 1970, the number of nurses on the staff rose to 23. This numerical improvement over the 1967 complement left the Unit qualitatively weaker. In 1967 not only the sisters but also the majority of the staff nurses were sufficiently experienced to take full responsibility in the ward. In 1970, apart from the 4 sisters on the permanent staff, all the nurses were under instruction. Because of the shortage of nurses fully trained in intensive care, these trainees had to accept periods of full responsibility in the ward during the second three months of their course. Unfortunately, on completion of their course very few stayed on as members of the permanent staff.

In 1974 staffing problems became so acute that at times it was possible to nurse only two patients at a time and total closure of the Unit seemed inevitable. For the first time since 1967 agency nurses, trained in intensive care, were employed during the greater part of the year as the number of trained permanent staff fell. Although the majority of these were capable of maintaining the expected high standard under supervision, few were considered competent to take charge of the Unit at night. Fortunately, 1975 saw an improvement in staffing in anticipation of the opening of the new 12-bedded Unit in 1976.

Student nurses in the intensive care unit

It has been said that an intensive care unit is no place for a student nurse. Nevertheless, all student nurses at Kingston Hospital spend six weeks in the Unit as part of their training; otherwise they would rarely see patients with acute myocardial infarction, those with a tracheostomy or those treated with mechanical artificial ventilation. Some have demonstrated an obvious aptitude for the work and are invited to join the training course after their State Registration. Familiarity with the Unit enables them to take responsibility earlier than those coming to take the course from other hospitals.

The use and abuse of the intensive care unit, 1967–75

It should be accepted that an intensive care unit is intended only for those patients whose treatment would benefit from its special facilities which are unobtainable in the general wards of the hospital. Nevertheless, a continuing administrative effort has been required to ensure that the Unit was used solely for the purpose for which it was established and that its services were not abused. This effort has been exercised in two directions; firstly, to limit the number of unnecessary admissions to the Unit and, secondly, to reduce unnecessarily prolonged bed occupancy when the need for intensive care had passed.

Factors affecting the numbers of admissions to the unit

Table 16.15 shows the total number of patients admitted in each triennium from 1967 to 1975 and the division of those patients into 'intensive care'

TABLE 16.15.   INTENSIVE CARE AND SHORT-STAY PATIENTS, 1967–75

	1967–69	1970–72	1973–75
Patients admitted	2 319	2 211	2 198
Intensive care patients	1 725	1 858	2 041
Short-stay patients	594	353	157
Short-stay other than circulatory disease	446	71	57

and 'short-stay' categories. The 'short-stay' category refers to those patients who, in retrospect, did not require the special facilities of the Unit. The years 1967–69 show the highest number of total admissions—2 319; but of these only 1 725 (74%) were for intensive care. There were 594 short-stay patients and thus 1967–69 can be regarded as the years of greatest abuse of the facilities of the Unit. The figures for succeeding years show the effect of efforts to curb this abuse. The years 1973–75 show the highest number of intensive care patients and the lowest frequency of admission of short-stay patients.

The number of short-stay patients should not necessarily be taken as an accurate indication of the extent to which the Unit has been misused. A considerable proportion of the patients in the Unit were suspected of suffering from myocardial infarction or other serious circulatory disease. A coronary care service implies the admission of all patients with suggestive symptoms in anticipation of a definitive diagnosis. Those patients who, after 24–48 hours' observation and investigation, were not proved to have serious circulatory disease were classified in the short-stay category. Consequently, a more accurate indication of the misuse of the unit should be measured by the total number of short-stay patients less those monitored for circulatory disease. The figures show a very drastic reduction since 1967–69.

Factors affecting bed occupancy in the unit

It is of particular importance that the nursing staff, never unduly numerous, should concentrate on patients genuinely in need of their attention and should not be distracted by patients with less urgent needs. The efficiency of an intensive care unit depends on the speed of diagnosis, effectiveness of treatment and the promptness of transfer to the general ward.

Table 16.16 gives some insight into the success of efforts to reduce unnecessary bed occupancy. In 1967–69, 1 725 intensive care patients occupied 5 879 patient-days or 3·41 days per patient. A gradual improvement over the years is suggested by the 1973–75 figures, which show 2 041 intensive care patients staying only 5 183 patient-days, or 2·54 days per patient. Thus, comparing 1967–69 with 1973–75, 316 more patients occupied 696 less days in the Unit. This may be due in part to the reduction in the number of patients with chronic lung disease with respiratory failure requiring long-term ventilator treatment. The number of long-stay

TABLE 16.16. BED OCCUPANCY BY INTENSIVE CARE PATIENTS

	1967–69	1970–72	1973–75
Total intensive care patients	1 725	1 858	2 041
Patient-days	5 879	5 380	5 183
Days per patient	3·41	2·90	2·54
Patients staying over 14 days in the Unit	52	26	26
Patients staying over 28 days in the Unit	8	5	2

patients, namely those remaining over 14 days in the Unit, fell from 52 in 1967–69 to 26 in 1970–72 and 1973–75. In the nine years 1967–75, out of a total of 104 long-stay patients, only 15 remained in the Unit for more than 28 days (Table 16.16).

It will be seen that this experience has differed from that of many other intensive care units in that the number of very long-stay patients has been small and few have ever appeared likely to occupy a bed in the Unit indefinitely.

Conclusions

The records suggest a very special gradual realization by the clinicians of the importance of using the intensive care unit intelligently and responsibly so that it can best fulfil its function. While this need may well be accepted by the consultant medical staff, the principles upon which the efficient practice of intensive care depend require frequent reiteration to the constantly changing junior medical staff in whose hands lies the immediate responsibility for the admission, care and transfer of individual patients. In making these somewhat critical comments, the writer is not unappreciative of the serious difficulties in maintaining high standards of patient care in the general wards of the hospital in the face of continuing acute shortage of beds and experienced nursing staff. It is, however, only by insulating the Unit from these pressures that the highest quality of intensive care can be maintained.

The anaesthetist and the intensive care unit

It has become customary in most hospitals to assign the task of administration of the intensive care unit to an anaesthetist. This is presumably so by the consent of his medical and surgical colleagues who see the anaesthetist's presumed clinical neutrality as an advantage on the rare occasions when he may have to arbitrate between the claims of patients for the scarce bed in the unit.

Anaesthetists readily accept involvement with intensive care, firstly because they see in it a widening of their clinical experience hitherto limited by the narrow confines of what goes on in an operating theatre, and secondly because they feel that they can make some contribution to the treatment of the patients by virtue of their specialized knowledge and practical expertise. It has never been the policy in this Unit for the anaesthetist to take total clinical charge of the patients who, in practice, remain under the control of the consultant in whose care they have been admitted. It can hardly be expected that an anaesthetist appointed in charge of an intensive care unit should be able to assume clinical responsibility for which he has neither the training, the experience nor the competence; in fact, the interests of some patients may best be served if he retains a healthy sense of his own limitations. Furthermore, an anaesthetist can hardly spend more than a small proportion of his clinical time in the intensive care unit if he is also heavily committed to his primary function, that of giving anaesthetics.

What, then, does the job involve? During nearly six years in the role of manager of the intensive care unit, the writer can say that it has included the following activities:

1. Formulation of the general policy concerning the use of the Unit and the services offered.

2. Assistance in the treatment of patients requiring resuscitation, ventilation and pain relief, and co-ordination of the treatment of patients with complex complaints involving more than one specialty.

3. Organization of the medical lectures given to nurses attending the course in intensive care, personally giving the majority of the lectures and giving informal bedside instruction to nurses on individual cases.

4. Maintaining a close liaison with the departmental sister-in-charge in the resolution of the problems affecting the efficient working of the Unit, and taking any action necessary to ensure that the facilities of the Unit are not misused.

5. Receiving and acting upon suggestions for the purchase of new equipment for the Unit.

6. Organization and supervision of the emergency resuscitation (Crash Call) system throughout the hospital.

7. Organization, maintenance and analysis of the records of patients treated in the Unit and the production of the Annual Report.

The job is therefore nebulous, but, apparently by common consent, necessary. It must be admitted that with the passing of time it has become less arduous and one can foresee that the need for a medical manager may no longer exist. Certainly that medical manager need not necessarily continue to be an anaesthetist. The technical dexterity involved in securing and maintaining a clear airway and an understanding of the inner working and peculiarities of mechanical ventilators need not remain his monopoly. Indeed, it has been argued that anaesthetists have become so involved with intensive care and emergency resuscitation that they cannot take on additional activities more specifically appropriate to the specialty of anaesthesia. In common with other hospital specialists, the anaesthetist would continue to serve the unit in helping with the treatment of patients and in the training of the nurses; but once an intensive care unit has been established and equipped and its therapeutic regimes standardized, his managerial functions could, and perhaps should, become redundant.

Index

Accurox, 49
Air embolus, 64
Airway pressure, 104
Airways resistance, 2
Alcohol (ethyl alcohol), 133
Alveolar air equation, 163
Alveolar CO_2, 169
Ambu bag, 101
Amino acid preparations, 134
Aminofusin, 135
Aminoplex, 135
Aminosol, 134
Anabolic phase, 129
Anaemic hypoxia, 44
Anaphylactic shock, 17
Anoxia, 44
Antibiotics, 185
Anxiety, 116
Aspiration secretions, 82
Asthma, 16
Astrup technique, 167
  apparatus, 166
Autoclavable circuits, 180
Automatic ventilators, 86
  choice of, 90, 101
  classification, 87
  disinfection, 179
  'fighting', 107
  ideal, 90
  motive force, 88
  paediatric, 144
  weaning off, 110

Bacterial filters, 180
Bacteriological monitoring, 184
Bladder—care of, 118
  aspiration of secretions, 81, 120
BLB mask, 48
Blease pulmoflator, 95
Bronchitis, 17
Blood–gas measurements, 29

Cape Bristol ventilator, 91
Cape multi-purpose ventilator, 91
Carbohydrate intake, 130, 131
Carbon dioxide—dissociation curve
  of, 4
Cardiac—arrest, 113
  output (effect on O_2 availability), 43
Cardiovascular disorders, 34
Casein hydrolysate (see also Aminosol),
  134
Catabolic phase, 129
Central nervous system depression, 10,
  32
Closing volume, 5
Collagen disease, 8
Compliance, 3
Complications of tracheostomy, 64
Condenser/humidifiers, 76
Continuous positive airway pressure
  (CPAP), 149
Coronary care in ICU, 195
Coughing, 81
Croup syndrome, 12
Cuff pressures, 61

Decannulation, 84
  in infants, 157
Diabetes, 139
Diet, 136
Diphtheria, 12
Disinfection, 177

East blower/humidifier, 77
East Radcliffe ventilator, 91
Elective tracheostomy, 53
Emphysema—subcutaneous, 66
Endotracheal intubation, 23
  in infants, 150
Engström ventilator, 95
Essential amino acids, 134
Ethylene oxide disinfection, 180

Examination of patient, 161
Eyes—care of, 118

Fats, 133
Fibrosing alveolitis, 8
Flow generator, 86
Forced expiratory volume (FEV_1), 2
Formaldehyde disinfection, 180

Granulomas of trachea, 69
Granulomatous lung lesions, 8
Growth hormone, 130

Haemorrhage, 64
Heated water reservoirs, 75, 77
Humidification, 75, 105
Hyperbaric oxygen, 51
Hypercarbia, 39
Hypocarbia, 39
Hypoglycaemia, 132
Hypoxaemia, 115
Hypoxia, 44
    assessment of, 45
    forms of, 115
Hypoxic drive, 46

Intensive Care Unit—admission to, 192
    nursing staff, 203
    place of anaesthetist, 206
    record card, 190
    special techniques, 194
    use and abuse of, 204
ICU in district general hospital, 189
Immunological factors, 172
Infection—causal organisms, 174
    control of, 175
    factors influencing, 170
    hospital-acquired, 171
    treatment of, 187
Infants and artificial ventilation, 143
Infection, 111, 170
Inhalation of vomit, 16
Insulin, 130
Intermittent mandatory ventilation (IMV), 109, 110
Intermittent positive pressure ventilation (IPPV), 38
    physiological effects of, 38
Isolation policy, 176

Kilopascal—SI units, 1

Laerdal bag, 101
Lanz tube, 36
Laryngeal inco-ordination, 68
Laryngeal oedema, 12
Laryngotomy, 23
    indication for, 22
Laryngo-tracheo-bronchitis, 12
Liver disease, 138
Lung function tests, 29

Magnesium, 137
Manley pulmovent, 99
MC oxygen mask, 48
Measurements—acid–base, 167
    alveolar CO_2, 169
    blood gases, 29, 166
    lung function, 29
    minute volume, 107
    significance, 161
    ventilation, 162
Microcirculation, 44
Minute volume, 107
Mixed venous oxygen content, 45
Mixomask, 49
Mouth—care of, 118
Multivent, 49
Muscle disorders, 11, 32

Narrow spectrum antibiotics, 186
Nebulizers, 75, 78
Neonates—artificial ventilation, 143
    tracheostomy, 143
Nursing—care of ventilated patient, 115
    schedule, 122
    services—organization, 121, 203
Nutrition, 110

Observations and records, 108, 116
Obstructive lung disease, 2, 33
Ohio gas nebulizer, 80
Organisms causing infection, 174
Oxyaire mask, 48
Oxygen—availability, 43, 105
    dissociation curve, 4, 41
    inspired concentration nomogram, 108
    tents, 50
    therapy, 19, 41, 47
    toxicity, 45, 144
    transport, 41

Paediatric ventilators, 144
Pain, 116

Parenteral nutrition, 129, 134
  indications for, 135
Patient—management of, 109
Patient-triggered ventilators, 109
Peak expiratory flow rate, 48
Perfusion of lung, 3
Peripheral nervous diseases, 11
Physiological dead space (*see also*
  Ventilation perfusion ratio), 37
Physiotherapy, 124–8
  aids, 126
  objectives, 124
  techniques, 125
Pink puffers, 9
Pneumask, 48
Pneumothorax, 11, 73
Poisoning, 200
  age distribution, 202
  poisons used, 201
  sex distribution, 202
  treatment of, 202
Polymask, 48
Portex tracheostomy tube, 36
Positive end-expiratory pressure
  (PEEP), 6, 38, 46, 149
Postoperative respiratory failure,
  20
Potassium, 137
Portogen mask, 48
Pressure areas, 119
Pressure generator, 86
Pressure-cycled ventilators, 87
Protein malnutrition, 129
Psychological care, 111, 121
Pulmonary compliance (*see also*
  Compliance), 3
Pulmonary embolus, 20
Pulmonary oxygen toxicity, 46

Records, 107, 116
Renal failure, 139
Residual volume, 3
Respiratory—depression, 46
  distress syndrome (adult), 14
    newborn, 13, 143
  failure, 1, 10, 198
    postoperative, 20
  insufficiency, 1
  intensive care, 198
    causes of, 199
  obstruction, 24
  stimulants, 18
Restrictive lung disease, 2, 33

Secretions—removal of, 81, 120
Shock lung, 14
Siemens Servo Ventilator, 97
Silent zone, 2
Sorbitol, 132
Statistical summary of ICU, Kingston
    Hospital, 191
Steam kettle, 78
Sterilization, 172
Subcutaneous emphysema, 66, 73
Subglottic oedema, 153
Subglottic stenosis, 153

Thyroid hormone, 130
Tidal volume, 104
Time cycling, 89
Total lung capacity, 2
Trace elements, 141
Trachea—damage, 68
  stenosis, 70
  ulceration, 69
Tracheitis, 65
Tracheomalacia, 69
Tracheo-oesophageal fistula, 71
Tracheostomy—care of, 119
  complications of, 64
  for prolonged ventilation, 26
  indication for, 22, 24
  in infants, 154
  infection in, 181
  management of, 74
  physiological effects, 36
  stoma, 57
  technique of performing, 53
  types of tracheostomy, 58
  types of tracheostomy tubes, 58
Tracheostomy tubes—blockage, 66
  changing, 83
  cuffs pressure, 61
  displacement of, 66, 73
  in infants, 155
  removal—decannulation, 84
  securing, 80
  types, 58
Travasol, 135
Trophysan, 135
Tunstall connector, 152

Ulceration of trachea, 69
Ultrasonic nebulizers, 78

Vamin, 135
Variomask, 49

Venepuncture, 182
Ventilation—control of, 106
Ventilation perfusion ratio, 4
Ventilators (*see also* Automatic ventilators), 86
  'fighting', 107
Ventimask, 19, 49

Venturi devices, 49
Vital capacity, 2
Vitamins, 141

Weaning from ventilator, 110
Wolfe bottle, 79
Wright respirometer, 101, 162